CASE STUDIES IN LIPID MANAGEMENT

CASE STUDIES IN LIPID MANAGEMENT

Edited by

D John Betteridge BSC MB PhD MD FRCP FAHA
Professor of Endocrinology and Metabolism
Division of Medicine
Royal Free and University College Medical School
London, UK

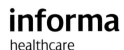

© 2007 Informa UK Ltd

First published in the United Kingdom in 2007 by Informa Healthcare, 4 Park Square, Milton Park, Abingdon, Oxon OX14 4RN. Informa Healthcare is a trading division of Informa UK Ltd. Registered Office: 37/41 Mortimer Street, London W1T 3JH. Registered in England and Wales Number 1072954.

Tel: +44 (0)20 7017 6000
Fax: +44 (0)20 7017 6699
Email: info.medicine@tandf.co.uk
Website: www.informahealthcare.com

A CIP record for this book is available from the British Library.
Library of Congress Cataloging-in-Publication Data

Data available on application

ISBN-10: 1 84184 477 2
ISBN-13: 978 1 84184 477 0

Distributed in North and South America by
Taylor & Francis
6000 Broken Sound Parkway, NW, (Suite 300)
Boca Raton, FL 33487, USA

Within Continental USA
Tel: 1 (800) 272 7737; Fax: 1 (800) 374 3401
Outside Continental USA
Tel: (561) 994 0555; Fax: (561) 361 6018
Email: orders@crcpress.com

Distributed in the rest of the world by
Thomson Publishing Services
Cheriton House
North Way
Andover, Hampshire SP10 5BE, UK
Tel: +44 (0)1264 332424
Email: tps.tandfsalesorder@thomson.com

Composition by C&M Digitals (P) Ltd, Chennai, India
Printed and bound in India by Replika Press Pvt. Ltd

CONTENTS

List of contributors   ix
Preface   xiii

Multiple risk factors

1. Moderate-risk patient with hypercholesterolemia:
   a pharmacy (P) model for decreasing LDL-cholesterol
   to reduce coronary heart disease risk   1
   Penny M Kris-Etherton and Thomas A Pearson

2. Targeting multiple lipid risk factors with combination
   lipid-lowering therapy to reduce cardiovascular risk   7
   Dean G Karalis

3. A lady with multiple risk factors
   for coronary heart disease   11
   Madhu Singh and David Nash

Patients with coronary heart disease

4. Coronary heart disease in a premenopausal woman   15
   Graham Jackson

5. Case study: women and cardiovascular risk   19
   James A Underberg

6. A patient with diabetes and coronary heart disease   23
   Mikko Syvänne

7. Lipid-modifying therapy in a person with
   diabetes and an acute coronary syndrome   29
   Andrew M Tonkin and Lei Chen

Severe dyslipidemias

8. A patient with the clinical phenotype of
   severe familial hypercholesterolemia   35
   Anton FH Stalenhoef

9. A case of successful treatment of
   familial hypercholesterolemia   39
   Anders G Olsson

10. LDL apheresis therapy during pregnancy   43
    Linda C Hemphill

11. A case of xanthomatous neuropathy   47
    Gilbert Thompson

12. Unusually severe dominant hypercholesterolemia   51
    Rossi Naoumova

13. A case of extreme triglyceridemia   55
    Richard L Dunbar

14. A patient with acute severe abdominal pain
    and generalized eruptive xanthomata   59
    Haralampos J Milionis and Moses S Elisaf

15. Severe hypertriglyceridemia due to familial
    lipoprotein lipase deficiency in pregnancy   65
    John R Burnett and Gerald F Watts

Combined hyperlipidemia

16. Managing combined hyperlipoproteinemia in a man with the
    metabolic syndrome   73
    Paul Nestel

17. Lipid therapy for dyslipidemia in the
    presence of the metabolic syndrome   79
    Sander J Robins

18. Familial combined hyperlipidemia:
    the case of triglycerides   85
    Manuel Castro Cabezas and Ton J Rabelink

19. Management of combined hyperlipidemia   95
    Philip J Barter

20. Fat in the liver: a feature of insulin resistance,
    dyslipidemia, and atherosclerosis?   99
    Dirk Müller-Wieland

21. Mixed lipemia with striking physical signs   105
    D John Betteridge

22. A case for measuring apoprotein B   109
    Beth Psaila and D John Betteridge

Secondary dyslipidemia

23. A hypercholesterolemic patient with
    hypothyroidism and something else   113
    Rafael Carmena and José T Real

24. Dry skin and cardiovascular health   117
    Ioanna Gouni-Berthold and Wilhelm Krone

25. Ethanol-induced combined hyperlipidemia   123
    Juhani Kahri and Marja Riitta-Taskinen

26. A patient with type 2 diabetes mellitus   127
    Kathryn CB Tan

27. A modicum of suspicion: diabetic kidney
    disease and dyslipidemia   131
    Merlin C Thomas and Per-Henrik Groop

28. A patient with peripheral arterial disease
    and metabolic syndrome   143
    Evangelos A Zacharis and Emmanuel S Ganotakis

29. A postmenopausal woman with marked hypertriglyceridemia   147
    Savitha Subramanian and Alan Chait

Therapeutic issues

30. Combination therapy of hyperlipidemia   153
    Henry N Ginsberg

vii

31. Use of combination therapy in a patient
    with complex dyslipidemia   159
    Peter P Toth and Michael H Davidson

32. Triple therapy in the treatment of hyperlipidemia   165
    Anthony S Wierzbicki

33. Grasping the nettle: the impact of
    lifestyle change in metabolic syndrome   171
    Maria Adiseshiah and D John Betteridge

34. A patient with dyslipidemia, coronary heart disease, and a history
    of statin intolerance   175
    Evangelos N Liberopoulos and Dimitri P Mikhailidis

35. Statin intolerance in a patient
    following a kidney transplant   179
    D John Betteridge

Contributors

Maria Adiseshiah RN MSc
Division of Medicine, Royal Free and
University College Medical School,
London, UK

Philip J Barter MD PhD
Director, The Heart Research
Institute, Camperdown, Sydney,
Australia

D John Betteridge BSc MB PhD MD
FRCP FAHA
Professor of Endocrinology and
Metablolism, Division of Medicine,
Royal Free and University College
Medical School,
London, UK

John R Burnett MD PhD FRCPA
Consultant Medical Biochemist,
Department of Core Clinical
Pathology & Biochemistry and Lipid
Disorders Clinic, Royal Perth
Hospital, and Clinical Associate
Professor, School of Medicine and
Pharmacology, University of
Western Australia, Perth, Australia

Manuel Castro Cabezas MD PhD
Department of Internal Medicine,
Center for Diabetes and Vascular
Medicine, St Franciscus Gasthuis,
Rotterdam, The Netherlands

Rafael Carmena MD
Endocrinology Service, University of
Valencia, Hospital Clinico
Universitario, Valencia, Spain

Alan Chait MD
Edwin L Bierman Professor of
Medicine, Head, Division of
Metabolism, Endocrinology and
Nutrition, Department of Medicine,
University of Washington,
Seattle, WA, USA

Lei Chen MD
NHMRC Clinical Centre of
Excellence and Therapeutics,
Department of Epidemiology
and Preventive Medicine, Monash
University, Melbourne, Victoria,
Australia

Michael H Davidson MD
Chicago Center for Clinical Research,
Director of Preventive Cardiology,
Rush Medical College,
Rush-Presbyterian-St
Luke's Medical Center,
Chicago, IL, USA

Richard L Dunbar MD
Instructor of Medicine, University of
Pennsylvania Medical School,
Philadelphia, PA, USA

Moses S Elisaf MD FRSH FASA
Professor of Medicine, Department of
Internal Medicine, University of
Ioannina, Ioannina, Greece

Emmanuel S Ganotakis MD
FRSH FASA
Assistant Professor of Medicine,
Department of Cardiology, University
Hospital of Crete, Heraklion, Greece

Henry N Ginsberg MD
Irving Professor of Medicine,
Director, Irving Center for Clinical
Research, Columbia University
College of Physicians and Surgeons,
New York, NY, USA

Ioanna Gouni-Berthold MD
Department of Internal Medicine II,
University of Cologne, Cologne,
Germany

Per-Henrik Groop MD DMSc
Director and Assistant Professor,
Folkhälsan Research Center,
Biomedicum Helsinki, University of
Helsinki, Helsinki, Finland

Linda C Hemphill MD
Massachusetts General Hospital,
Cardiology Department, Boston, MA,
USA

Graham Jackson FRCP FESC FACC
Guy's and St Thomas' NHS Trust, UK

Juhani Kahri MD PhD
Department of Internal Medicine,
Division of Cardiology, Helsinki
University Central Hospital, Helsinki,
Finland

Dean G Karalis MD FACC
Clinical Associate Professor
of Medicine, Drexel University
College of Medicine,
Philadelphia, PA, USA

Penny M Kris-Etherton PhD RD
Distinguished Professor of Nutrition,
Department of Nutritional Sciences,
The Pennsylvania State University,
University Park, PA, USA

Wilhelm Krone MD
Department of Internal Medicine II,
University of Cologne, Cologne,
Germany

Evagelos N Liberopoulos MD FASA
Research Fellow, Department of
Clinical Biochemistry (Lipid Clinics),
Royal Free Hospital and University
College Medical School,
London, UK

Dimitri P Mikhailidis BSc MSc MD
FACB FASA FFPM FRCP FRCPath
Reader and Honorary Consultant,
Academic Head of Department,
Department of Clinical Biochemistry
(Lipid Clinics), Royal Free Hospital
and University College Medical
School, London, UK

Haralampos J Milionis MD
Lecturer in Internal Medicine,
Department of Internal Medicine,
School of Medicine, University of
Ioannina, Greece

Dirk Müller-Wieland MD
Deutsches Diabetes-Zentrum,
Düsseldorf, Germany

Rossi Naoumova MD PhD MRCP FAHA
MRC Senior Clinical Scientist/Hon
Consultant Physician in Lipidology,
Lipid Clinic, Hammersmith Hospital,
London, UK

David Nash MD MBA
Jefferson University, Department of
Health Policy, Philadelphia, PA, USA

Paul Nestel MD
Professor, Cardiovascular Nutrition
Laboratory and Alfred & Baker
Medical Unit, Baker Medical Research
Institute, Melbourne, Australia

Anders G Olsson MD PhD
Professor of Internal Medicine,
Department of Medicine and Care,
Berzelius Science Park, University
Hospital, Linköping, Sweden

Thomas A Pearson MD MPH PhD
Department Chair and Albert D
Kaiser Professor, Department of
Community and Preventive Medicine,
Division of Epidemiology, University
of Rochester, Rochester, NY, USA

Beth Psaila MRCP
Division of Medicine, Royal Free and
University College Medical School,
London, UK

Ton J Rabelink PhD
Head, Department of Nephrology,
LUMC Leiden, The Netherlands

José T Real MD
Endocrinology Service, Hospital
Clinico Universitario, Valencia, Spain

Marja Riitta-Taskinen MD PhD
Department of Internal Medicine,
Division of Cardiology, Helsinki
University Central Hospital,
Finland

Sander J Robins MD
Laboratory Director, Framingham
Heart Study Professor of Medicine,
Boston University School of Medicine,
Boston, MA, USA

Madhu Singh MD MRCP
Outcomes Research Fellow,
Thomas Jefferson University,
Department of Health Policy,
Philadelphia, PA, USA

Anton FH Stalenhoef MD PhD FRCP
Professor of Medicine, Department of
Medicine, Radboud University
Nijmegen Medical Centre,
Nijmegen, The Netherlands

Savitha Subramanian MD
Head, Division of Metabolism,
Endocrinology and Nutrition,
Department of Medicine,
University of Washington Seattle,
WA, USA

Mikko Syvänne MD PhD
Associate Professor, Division of
Cardiology, Helsinki University
Central Hospital,
Helsinki, Finland

Kathryn CB Tan MBBCH MD
Associate Professor, Department of
Medicine, Queen Mary Hospital,
Hong Kong

xi

Merlin C Thomas MD
Associate Professor of Epidemiology,
Department of Epidemiology,
Monash University, AMREP Precinct,
Melbourne, Victoria, Australia

Gilbert Thompson
Emeritus Professor of Clinical
Lipidology, Department of Metabolic
Medicine, Imperial College,
Hammersmith Hospital,
London, UK

Andrew M Tonkin MD FRACP
NHMRC Centre of Clinical Research
Excellence in Therapeutics,
Department of Epidemiology
and Preventive Medicine,
Monash University,
Victoria, Australia

Peter P Toth MD PhD FAAFP FICA FAHA
FCCP FACC
Director of Preventive Cardiology,
Sterling Rock Falls Clinic Sterling, IL
and Chief of Medicine, CGH Medical
Center, Clinical Associate Professor,
University of Illinois School of
Medicine, IL, USA

James A Underberg MS MD
Preventive Cardiovascular Medicine,
Diplomate, American Board of Clinical
Lipidology and Clinical Assistant
Professor of Medicine, Division of
General Internal Medicine, NYU
Medical School, NY, USA

Gerald F Watts DSC MD PhD FRACP
Consultant Physician, Department of
Internal Medicine and Lipid Disorders
Clinic, Royal Perth Hospital and
Professor, School of Medicine and
Pharmacology, University of Western
Australia, Perth, Australia

Anthony S Wierzbicki DM DPhil
FRCPath FAHA
Consultant Chemical Pathologist,
St Thomas's Hospital, London, UK

Evangelos A Zacharis MD
Senior Registrar, Department of
Cardiology, University Hospital of
Crete, Heraklion Greece

PREFACE

Over the last decade or so the impressive data accumulated from controlled clinical endpoint trials have moved lipid management center stage in many areas of medicine. Routine management of lipid disorders has moved from lipid clinics into primary care and many other specialist clinics such as cardiology, diabetology, neurology, and nephrology. Furthermore, the emphasis in many individual patients is the identification and management of overall cardiovascular risk.

Given the impressive safety database, particularly for the statins, many physicians now feel confident in the use of these drugs in the majority of their patients. Increasingly lipid specialists are only referred more complex secondary or familial dyslipidemias or patients where first-line therapy has failed or has not been tolerated. Hopefully this book of cases will provide the interested physician with the shared clinical experience of experts in the field which they can utilize in their own practice.

I have approached highly experienced international colleagues to present cases that they have found fascinating and have learned from. In my experience physicians thoroughly enjoy the learning experience gained from case discussions. The cases do not cover the whole of the subject but certainly reflect many of the interesting clinical challenges currently faced. They should provide 'instant' experience not only for colleagues in other specialities but also those primarily interested in lipid metabolism.

I would like to thank my colleagues and friends for their contributions to this book, their enthusiasm for the project, and their willingness to pass on their experience.

My publishers and in particular Alan Burgess and Lindsay Campbell have been very supportive and patient. As always I and my colleagues should thank our patients who continue to inspire and challenge us to greater efforts in clinical management and research.

D John Betteridge

Case 1

MODERATE-RISK PATIENT WITH HYPERCHOLESTEROLEMIA: A PHARMACY (P) MODEL FOR DECREASING LDL-CHOLESTEROL TO REDUCE CORONARY HEART DISEASE RISK

Penny M Kris-Etherton and Thomas A Pearson

Introduction

Cardiovascular diseases (CVD) are a leading cause of death in the UK. Coronary heart disease, the most prevalent CVD, accounts for 117000 deaths yearly in the UK. Moreover, almost 270000 individuals have a heart attack annually, and approximately 30% die before reaching health-care facilities. Priorities for CHD prevention in clinical practice are for patients with CHD or other major atherosclerotic disease. In addition, patients with diabetes are also a high-risk group. Major risk factors for CHD include cigarette smoking, an elevated LDL-cholesterol level (> 3.0 mmol/l), elevated blood pressure (systolic blood pressure $\geq$ 140 mm Hg; diastolic blood pressure $\geq$ 85 mm Hg), family history of premature CHD (CHD in male first degree relatives < 55 years; CHD in female first degree relatives < 65 years), and age (men $\geq$ 45 years; women $\geq$ 55 years). The ratio of serum total cholesterol to HDL-cholesterol is used to assess coronary risk; therefore, low HDL-cholesterol contributes to increased risk. The Joint British Societies have developed coronary risk prediction charts for men and women (smoking vs nonsmoking status) that are primarily linked to systolic blood pressure, and the ratio of serum total cholesterol to HDL-cholesterol, and stratified by age.

There is an impressive database that demonstrates the benefits of decreasing CHD risk factors on CHD morbidity and mortality. One major risk factor that has been the target of intervention efforts is an elevated LDL-cholesterol level. Both primary and secondary prevention studies have clearly shown that decreasing LDL-cholesterol level reduces coronary event rates. For every 1% decrease in

LDL-cholesterol, risk for hard CHD events (myocardial infarction and CHD death) is decreased by approximately 1%. Studies that induced a more prolonged reduction in LDL-cholesterol have been shown to evoke an even greater reduction in CHD risk.

Diet and physical activity continue to be the first line of therapy for treating an elevated LDL-cholesterol level. The recommended diet is high in fruits, vegetables, whole grains, lean protein foods (i.e. low-fat dairy products, meats, and poultry), and includes two portions of fish per week, one of which should be oily. In addition, achieving and maintaining a healthy body weight (a BMI between 19 and 24.9 kg/m^2) is a goal that beneficially affects LDL-cholesterol as well as other CHD risk factors. Moderate physical activity (approximately 30 minutes daily, most days of the week) also is recommended. An LDL-cholesterol-lowering diet that includes viscous fiber (5–10 g/day) and plant sterols/stanols (2 g/day) can reduce LDL-cholesterol as much as 20–30%. Frequently, the LDL-cholesterol goal is not achieved by lifestyle interventions.

Pharmacologic therapy is an important adjunctive intervention for achieving LDL-cholesterol goals as a means to reduce risk of CHD. The management of some conditions with non-prescription pharmacologic agents is being considered, and even implemented. Symptomatic conditions, such as headache, heartburn, etc., have been the basis for non-pharmacologic therapy, including aspirin and antacids. However, there has been a shift in thinking about using non-pharmacologic therapy for some asymptomatic conditions. Examples of this include: inhibition of pancreatic lipase secretion (to block fat absorption) to facilitate weight loss (in the US); reduction of LDL-cholesterol level using a statin drug (in the UK). The statin drugs have become the primary pharmacologic intervention for lowering LDL-cholesterol levels, and in all countries with the exception of the UK, these are regulated as a prescription drug. In the UK, however, a 10 mg statin dose is available as a pharmacy-only 'P' medicine that is sold only from registered pharmacies under the supervision of a pharmacist. The intent of the 'P' program is to establish a new standard of communication that educates, supports, and motivates individuals to address not only an elevated LDL-cholesterol but also all other modifiable CHD risk factors. This program is intended for individuals who are at moderate risk of CHD. Moderate risk (approximately 10–15% 10-year risk of a first major coronary event) as determined by JBS Guidelines 1998 is defined as men >45 years of age or women aged 55 years or more with one or more of the following risk factors: first degree relative (parent or sibling) younger than 55 years for men or 65 years for women with a history of CHD; smoker (is currently a smoker or has been a smoker in the past 12 months); overweight/obese (BMI>25 kg/m^2) or truncal obesity (waist:

≥ 102 cm in men; ≥ 88 cm in women); South Asian ethnicity (Indian subcontinent). For the 'P' medicine program, the risk estimation is determined by assuming age-specific population means for total cholesterol/HDL-cholesterol levels, and blood pressure. Based on an extensive literature, 10 mg simvastatin per day reduces LDL-cholesterol by as much as
30%. Accordingly, this would be expected to reduce the risk of CHD by about 30%. In a 10–15% 10-year risk population, a 30% relative risk reduction is equivalent to an absolute risk reduction of between 3 and 5%.

Case study

A 47-year-old man comes to your office for a routine physical exam. He is in good health and his BMI is 25 kg/m^2. During his visit he asks your opinion about the 'P' medicine statin drug program for lowering his LDL-cholesterol level. He is concerned because his brother (age 51 years) has just been diagnosed with angina. Your patient has two children (16 and 17 years) who are eager to attend college. A successful businessman who owns a small company that is rapidly growing; your patient has many job-related demands. He shares a concern about having a fatal heart attack in the near future. Because your patient is a 'hard-charging' executive he wants to take control of his health. He wants to do anything he can to decrease his risk of CHD. Your patient does not smoke cigarettes, has a sedentary lifestyle, follows a diet that lacks recommended amounts of fruits and vegetables (five to nine servings/day) and whole grains (three servings/day), and is high in fatty meats and full-fat dairy products. He drinks alcohol in moderation. His blood pressure is normal (122/80) and based on last year's lipid profile, his total cholesterol was 5.8 mmol/l and his HDL-cholesterol was 1.3 mmol/l.

Questions

1. What would you advise this patient about taking this 'P' medicine statin drug?
2. What other recommendations would you make about lifestyle interventions that your patient could implement to decrease CHD risk?
3. What follow-up recommendations would you make, assuming that he follows your advice?

Further reading

Baigent C, Keech A, Kearney PM et al., and Cholesterol Treatment Trialists' (CTT) Collaborators. Efficacy and safety of cholesterol-lowering treatment: prospective meta-analysis of data from 90,056 participants in 14 randomised trials of statins. Lancet 2005; 366: 1267–78.

British Cardiac Society, British Hyperlipidaemia Association, British Hypertension Society, and British Diabetic Association. Joint British recommendations on prevention of coronary heart disease in clinical practice: Summary. BMJ 2000; 320: 705–8.

Jackson R, Lawes CM, Bennett DA, Milne RJ, Rodgers A. Treatment with drugs to lower blood pressure and blood cholesterol based on an individual's absolute cardiovascular risk. Lancet 2005; 365: 434–41.

Kris-Etherton PM, Harris WS, Appel LJ, and American Heart Association Nutrition Committee. Fish consumption, fish oil, omega-3 fatty acids, and cardiovascular disease. Circulation 2002; 106: 2747–57.

McKenney JM (ed.). Report of the National Lipid Association's Statin Safety Task Force. Am J Cardiol 2006; 97: Suppl S1.

Meilin JM, Struble WE, Tipping RW et al. A consumer use study of over-the-counter lovastatin (CUSTOM). Am J Cardiol 2004; 94: 1243–8.

Pearson TA. Population benefits of cholesterol reduction: Epidemiology, economics, and ethics. Am J Cardiol 2000; 85: 20E–23E

Pearson RA. The undertreatment of LDL-cholesterol: Addressing the challenge. Int J Cardiol 2000; Suppl 1: S23–S28.

Pearson TA. The epidemiologic basis for population-wide cholesterol reduction in the primary prevention of coronary disease. Am J Cardiol 2004; 94: 4F–8F

Sundquist K, Qvist J, Johansson SE, Sundquist J. The long-term effect of physical activity on incidence of coronary heart disease: a 12-year follow-up study. Prev Med 2005; 41: 219–25.

United Kingdom Scientific Advisory Committee on Nutrition. Paper FICS/04/02. March, 2004.

Answers

1. The patient meets the criteria for enrolling in the 'P' medicine statin program, and should be encouraged to participate in this program to decrease his risk of CHD.

You should recommend that he follow all product instructions. Your patient is classified at moderate risk for CHD because of his gender and age (> 45 years), and the presence of one additional risk factor — family history of premature CHD. The 10 mg dose of simvastatin would be expected to lower his LDL-cholesterol by 30%. His LDL-cholesterol is 3.48 mmol/l. Consequently, with a 30% reduction, his LDL-cholesterol would be 2.44 mmol/l. After treatment, his total cholesterol would be about 4.06 mmol/l and his total cholesterol:HDL-cholesterol ratio would be 3.1. NOTE: the recommendations of the JBC for total cholesterol and LDL-cholesterol are < 5 mmol/l and 3 mmol/l, respectively.

2. The patient should follow a heart healthy diet that includes fruits and vegetables, whole grains, low-fat dairy products, and lean protein sources. It would be appropriate to recommend consumption of sterol/stanol ester-containing products (i.e. margarine) that provide 2 g/day. In addition, the patient should be advised to consume food sources of viscous fiber (10–25 g/day). Two servings of fish (preferably oily) per week are recommended. The patient should be advised to participate in 30 minutes of moderate intensity physical activity most days of the week. These lifestyle interventions would be expected to further reduce total and LDL-cholesterol beyond that achieved with a 10 mg statin dose. The program of physical activity may increase HDL-cholesterol, and thus modify the total cholesterol to HDL-cholesterol ratio beyond that attained via the statin drug and cholesterol-lowering diet.

3. Although muscle myopathy is very rare, especially for a 10 mg/day dose of a statin drug, the patient should be advised to note if any muscle pain, tenderness, or weakness occurs. There is little to no hepatic risk at this statin dose for patients with normal hepatic function. To monitor the effects of the statin drug and lifestyle intervention program, the patient should be encouraged to have his blood cholesterol levels monitored, at which time liver function could be assessed.

Case 2

Targeting Multiple Lipid Risk Factors With Combination Lipid-Lowering Therapy To Reduce Cardiovascular Risk

Dean G Karalis

Case report

A 69-year-old man with a history of hypertension and coronary heart disease (CHD) developed symptoms of exertional angina. He had undergone coronary artery bypass surgery 8 years earlier. He had smoked cigarettes but quit at the time of his cardiac surgery. A recent myocardial perfusion stress test revealed ischemia in the anterior wall at a high exercise workload. Cardiac catheterization revealed severe native coronary artery disease. The left internal mammary to the left anterior descending coronary artery was occluded as was the saphenous vein graft to the right coronary artery. A sequential saphenous vein graft to the first and second marginal branches was widely patent and collaterals from the left circumflex coronary artery supplied the native distal left anterior descending and right coronary arteries.

The patient was treated medically for his angina with atenolol 50 mg daily and enteric coated aspirin, 325 mg daily. He was on no lipid-lowering therapy and simvastatin 40 mg a day was started. He did well for the next 3 years but again developed recurrent symptoms of exertional angina. A repeat myocardial perfusion stress test revealed worsening ischemia in the anterior wall and new ischemia in the inferior wall. In contrast to his previous stress test the ischemia this time developed at a low exercise workload. Cardiac catheterization now revealed severe disease in the saphenous vein graft to both marginal branches. He underwent repeat coronary artery bypass surgery, after which his angina was relieved.

Following surgery he was maintained on simvastatin at a dose of 40 mg a day and referred to our clinic for further evaluation and lipid management. On physical exam he weighed 190 pounds and had a waist circumference of 38 inches. His seated blood pressure measured 130/80 mm Hg. There was a 2/6 systolic ejection murmur heard loudest at the left sternal border. His physical exam was otherwise unremarkable. Six months after his second coronary bypass surgery his

7

Table 1 Lipid profile

Lipids	Baseline	On simvastatin 40 mg / day	On simvastatin 40 mg/day and extended-release niacin 2g /day
Total cholesterol (mg/dl)	227	175	142
Triglycerides (mg/dl)	203	191	122
LDL-cholesterol (mg/dl)	151	101	73
HDL-cholesterol (mg/dl)	35	36	45

lipid levels on 40 mg of simvastatin were as follows: total cholesterol 175 mg/dl, triglycerides 191 mg/dl, LDL-cholesterol 101 mg/dl, and HDL-cholesterol 36 mg/dl. The rest of the laboratory values were normal. He was counseled on lifestyle modification and prescribed a low-fat diet and an exercise regimen. Simvastatin was continued and extended-release niacin was started at a dose of 500 mg daily and slowly titrated up to a total of 2 g a day. He was also started on 2 g of fish oil tablets daily. No skin flushing or other side effects occurred as the dose of niacin was titrated up. On follow-up he had lost 12 pounds. With lifestyle modification and combination lipid-lowering therapy his lipid profile improved, with a marked increase in his HDL-cholesterol and further decrease in his LDL-cholesterol and triglyceride levels (Table 1). Now 5 years after his second coronary artery bypass procedure he remains angina-free and is doing well.

Discussion

Patients with CHD are at risk of recurrent cardiovascular events. Over the last decade several large randomized clinical trials with statin therapy have shown that lowering LDL-cholesterol with a statin can significantly reduce cardiovascular risk in these patients. Current guidelines for patients with CHD recommend lowering LDL-cholesterol to < 100 mg/dl with an optional goal of < 70 mg/dl in those patients at the highest risk.[1] Despite the reductions in cardiovascular morbidity and mortality seen with statin therapy, patients treated with statins remain at risk for progressive coronary artery disease and recurrent cardiovascular events. Recent attention has focused on targeting other lipid risk factors such as low levels of HDL-cholesterol and high levels of triglycerides once the primary target of LDL-cholesterol lowering with a statin has been met.

In the present case LDL-cholesterol was lowered to goal with statin therapy, yet the patient developed progressive coronary atherosclerosis and required repeat coronary artery bypass surgery. When the clinician is faced with such a patient, one treatment option would be to lower LDL-cholesterol further to < 70 mg/dl. Observational studies suggest that the lower the level of LDL-cholesterol, the lower the cardiovascular risk. In the recent Treat to New Targets study[2] over 10 000 patients with CHD whose LDL-cholesterol was at goal on atorvastatin 10 mg daily (mean LDL-cholesterol level of 98 mg/dl) were randomized to either stay on this dose or take a higher dose of atorvastatin, 80 mg daily. In the high-dose atorvastatin group LDL-cholesterol was lowered to 77 mg/dl, an additional 21% reduction. Those patients randomized to high-dose atorvastatin had a 24% lower risk of major cardiovascular events and a 25% lower risk of stroke compared with patients in the low-dose atorvastatin group. Compared to the low dose, 80 mg of atorvastatin was well tolerated. There was no increased risk of serious myopathy and only an additional 1% increase in the risk of developing significant elevation in liver function tests. The investigators in this study concluded that patients with CHD would benefit from more aggressive LDL-cholesterol lowering to levels lower than currently recommended.

Another treatment option in this patient would be to target his low level of HDL-cholesterol. Long-term observational studies have shown that the lower the HDL-cholesterol the higher the risk of cardiovascular disease. Current guidelines do not recommend a specific target level of HDL-cholesterol, but do recommend that physicians consider treating high-risk patients with medications to raise HDL-cholesterol. Although statins will raise HDL-cholesterol by a small degree, the most potent agent available to raise HDL-cholesterol is niacin. Niacin can raise HDL-cholesterol by 20–30%, lower triglycerides by up to 30%, and lower LDL-cholesterol by up to 20%.[3] Most of the benefit of raising HDL-cholesterol and lowering triglyceride levels occurs at the lower dose of niacin (1 g). At this dose little change in LDL-cholesterol occurs. The LDL-cholesterol-lowering properties of niacin are seen at higher doses (2 g). In the present case, the addition of 2 g of extended-release niacin raised HDL-cholesterol by 25%. Triglyceride levels fell by 19% and LDL-cholesterol fell to 73 mg/dl, an additional 28% reduction.

The main side effect of niacin is skin flushing. Although skin flushing occurs in most patients, the episodes of flushing are typically mild and do not necessitate stopping the medication. Extended-release preparations of niacin have been associated with less flushing. Flushing can be further reduced by dosing the extended-release niacin at bedtime and by premedicating with aspirin. Liver function studies need to be followed as the niacin dose is up-titrated and patients need to be counseled on the signs and symptoms of myopathy, although this latter complication is extremely rare. Although studies have shown a reduction in cardiovascular event rate and mortality with niacin in patients with CHD, large randomized trials comparing the combination of statin and niacin to statin alone are lacking. A recent small study[4] randomized 167 patients with stable coronary artery disease and low levels of HDL-cholesterol to statin alone or statin in combination with extended-release niacin (1 g daily). The treated LDL-cholesterol in the statin alone group was 86 mg/dl, within guideline goals. Niacin raised HDL-cholesterol by 21% and was well tolerated. No patient developed myopathy or significant elevation in liver function tests. In this study combination statin and niacin therapy reduced the progression of carotid wall thickening by 68% at 1 year compared with statin therapy alone.

This case illustrates that combination lipid-lowering therapy can be used safely in high-risk patients to target multiple lipid abnormalities. When niacin was added to statin therapy in this patient not only did the levels of HDL-cholesterol rise, but levels of triglycerides and LDL-cholesterol were further lowered. Combination therapy should be employed more often in high-risk patients to achieve optimal lipid levels. Ongoing studies will help determine if this strategy will reduce the risk of recurrent cardiovascular events and cardiovascular death in patients with CHD.

References

1. Grundy SM, Cleeman JI, Bairey Merz N et al. Implications of recent clinical trials for the National Cholesterol Education Program Adult Treatment Panel III guidelines. Circulation 2004; 110: 227–39.
2. LaRosa JC, Grundy SM, Waters DD et al. Intensive lipid lowering with atorvastatin in patients with stable coronary disease. N Engl J Med 2005; 352: 1425–35.
3. Wolfe ML, Vartanian SF, Ross JL et al. Safety and effectiveness of *Niaspan* when added sequentially to a statin for treatment of dyslipidemia. Am J Cardiol 2001; 87: 476–9.
4. Taylor AJ, Sullenberger LE, Lee HJ, Lee JK, Grace KA. Arterial biology for the investigation of the treatment effects of reducing cholesterol (ARBITER) 2. A double-blind, placebo-controlled study of extended-release niacin on atherosclerosis progression in secondary prevention patients treated with statins. Circulation 2004; 110: 3512–17.

Case 3

A Lady With Multiple Risk Factors For Coronary Heart Disease

Madhu Singh and David Nash

A 53-year-old woman saw her primary care physician for follow-up of treatment of hypercholesterolemia after she had relocated to a different part of the country. She gave a diagnosis of having 'high cholesterol' since the age of 41. Her hypercholesterolemia was treated only after she suffered a myocardial infarction a year later. For her coronary disease she underwent coronary artery bypass grafting (CABG) to repair two blood vessels. Three years after her CABG she needed single vessel coronary stenting.

Her initial treatment for hyperlipidemia was with lovastatin 20 mg/day, which she could not tolerate for longer than a year because of muscle aches. Subsequently she was started on gemfibrozil 600 mg twice a day, which she tolerated for about a year but she was switched to simvastatin 40 mg/day due to perceived poor response to gemfibrozil. She did not get a good enough response to escalating dosage with simvastatin so she was changed to atorvastatin 60 mg/day. According to the patient herself, her lipid panel improved somewhat on this therapy, but was far from normal.

The blood tests that she provided to her new primary care doctor were as follows, November 2000:

- Triglycerides 286 mg/dl
- Total cholesterol 332 mg/dl
- HDL-cholesterol 51 mg/dl
- LDL-cholesterol 224 mg/dl.

At this point in time, she was started on nicotinic acid, which she could not tolerate because of flushing.

Lipid panel September 2001:

- Triglyceride 405 mg/dl
- Total cholesterol 297 mg/dl
- HDL-cholesterol 44 mg/dl
- LDL-cholesterol values not calculated because of high triglyceride levels.

11

Next year in May 2003 her numbers had not changed substantially but she was now diagnosed to be diabetic with HbA1c of 8.1.

- Triglycerides 431 mg/dl
- Total cholesterol 247 mg/dl
- HDL-cholesterol 40 mg/dl.

At this time she was on atorvastatin 60 mg/day, which according to her was effective therapy; although causing her a lot of myalgia. Her current lipid panel is:

- Triglycerides 494 mg/dl
- Total cholesterol 219 mg/dl
- HDL-cholesterol 42 mg/dl.

Her liver function test done at the same time gave the following values: ALT 65, AST 49, alkaline phosphatase 215. Her thyroid function tests are normal. She is now on a combination of ezetimibe/simvastatin 10 mg/40 mg daily.

She is presently asymptomatic for cardiac complaints, although she feels tired all the time. Her father died when he was 50 years old of a myocardial infarction. Her mother lived to be 80 years old and died after a stroke. She is menopausal and complains bitterly of hot flashes and insomnia. She has been a lifelong nonsmoker and consumes wine occasionally.

On physical examination her body weight is 204 lbs, height 5'8", BMI 32, waist circumference 38", blood pressure 110/75, and pulse 68 regular. She says she has lost 10 lbs over the past 6 months on the basis of diet and exercise. She has no xanthomas.

Going over her blood results a presumptive diagnosis of familial combined hyperlipidemia was made.

Issues

This case study raises several questions – the initial lipid management was suboptimal. This may be due to physician or patient factors.

Her diagnosis of familial combined hyperlipidemia puts her at clearly increased risk of coronary heart disease (CHD).[1] In addition to a direct role in atherogenesis, hypertriglyceridemia tends to be associated with other abnormalities like low levels of HDL-cholesterol,[2] presence of small dense LDL particles, presence of atherogenic triglyceride-rich lipoprotein remnants, insulin resistance,[3] and increases in coagulability and viscosity.[4] According to her examination and blood results she fulfills the criteria for metabolic syndrome.

Her therapy should be intensified to include gemfibrozil to raise HDL-cholesterol levels and decrease triglyceride levels.[5] She did not tolerate niacin, which would have been a useful addition, although it could potentially worsen diabetic control. She has tried a variety of lipid-lowering agents and it may be helpful now to think about fish oil supplements,[6] which can lower serum triglyceride concentration by more than 50%. However, this may increase LDL-cholesterol levels so should be used in severe hypertriglyceridemia only.[7] The goal in her case should be to lower LDL-cholesterol to at least 100 mg/dl and maybe even 70 mg/dl.[8] This intensive approach can only work if she is an active participant in her care and understands the need for therapy. Statins are indicated in her therapy to reduce LDL-cholesterol levels, but fibrates and nicotinic acid are the most effective triglyceride-lowering drugs and have the added benefit of increasing HDL-cholesterol levels. Other risk factors also need to be addressed – weight loss, diabetic control, and hypertension. In her case, for optimal cardiovascular health, a lot of work lies ahead.

References

1. Cullen P. Evidence that triglycerides are an independent coronary heart disease risk factor. Am J Cardiol 2000; 86: 943–9.
2. Wittrup HH, Tybjaerg-Hansen A, Nordestgaard BG. Lipoprotein lipase mutations, plasma lipids and lipoproteins, and risk of ischemic heart disease. A meta-analysis. Circulation 1999; 99: 2901–7.
3. DeFronzo RA, Ferrannin E. Insulin resistance. A multifaceted syndrome responsible for NIDDM, obesity, hypertension, dyslipidemia, and atherosclerotic cardiovascular disease. Diabetes Care 1991; 14: 173–94.
4. Simpson HCR, Meade TW, Stirling Y et al. Hypertriglyceridemia and hypercoagulability. Lancet 1983; 1: 786–90.
5. Rubins HB, Robins SJ, Collins D et al., for the Veterans Affairs High-Density Lipoprotein Cholesterol Intervention Trial Study Group. Gemfibrozil for the secondary prevention of coronary heart disease in men with low levels of HDL-C. N Engl J Med 1999; 341: 410–18.
6. Durrington PN, Bhatnagar D, Mackness MI et al. An omega-3 polyunsaturated fatty acid concentrate administered for one year decreased triglycerides in simvastatin treated patients with coronary heart disease and persistent hypertriglyceridemia. Heart 2001; 85: 544–8.
7. Pharmaceutical Approvals monthly. F-D-C Reports. Chevy Chase, MD 2005; 10(2): 34.
8. Executive Summary of the Third Report of the NCEP Expert Panel on Detection, Evaluation and Treatment of High Blood Cholesterol in Adults. JAMA 2001; 285: 2486–97.

Case 4

CORONARY HEART DISEASE IN A PREMENOPAUSAL WOMAN

Graham Jackson

Introduction

The increasing incidence of coronary artery disease (CAD) in women and its often atypical presentation mean that as a profession we need to be alert to the possibility of CAD even in younger women.[1] In addition, a good history in an unlikely individual should not be dismissed, especially in the presence of recognized risk factors.

The case

A 43-year-old premenopausal Afro-Caribbean lady with hypertension was referred by her family doctor. She had just registered with the practice and was taking lisinopril 15 mg daily but her blood pressure was poorly controlled at 160/110 mm Hg. The doctor added atenolol 100 mg daily and the pressure improved to 140/102 mm Hg. Her renal function was normal and the fasting cholesterol was 5.8 mmol/l, triglycerides 1.0, HDL-cholesterol 2.7, and LDL-cholesterol 2.6 mmol/l. Her hemoglobin was 15.6 g/dl and glucose 4.7 mmol/l. She was complaining of chest tightness 'on and off' for a year, which she was not unduly concerned about. A trial of glyceryl trinitrate sublingually had surprisingly been beneficial. When I saw her I noted that she was overweight with a body mass index (BMI) of 30 kg/m^2 and had been smoking 10 cigarettes a day. Her resting ECG was normal. Her echocardiogram showed mild left ventricular hypertrophy and good left ventricular function.

So here was a most unlikely candidate for CAD – her history she played down, her lipids were reassuring regarding her HDL and LDL levels and she was the wrong age, gender, and racial group. Could this all be hypertension which needed better control and the use of a calcium antagonist as per the British Hypertension Society Guidelines for people of this racial origin? Experience has taught me to pursue the chest pain story in women no matter how atypical it can appear.

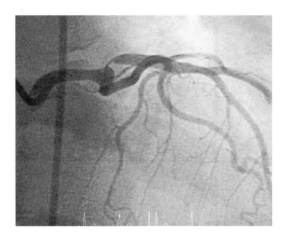

Figure 1   *Severe osteal left anterior descending stenosis.*

In doing so she admitted that the tightness across the chest was on occasion exercise-related, particularly steep hills, and was relieved by rest. It also occurred when stressed at work (she has a responsible job in the financial world) or over-excited and it had radiated to both arms, the left more than the right. Against her wishes ('can't you just change the drugs?') I organized an exercise ECG, expecting to establish hypertension rather than ischemia as the cause of her symptoms. To my surprise and concern she only managed 4 minutes on the treadmill when she developed her typical chest tightness, and also anterior ST elevation, suggesting a significant proximal left coronary lesion. Her blood pressure was 150/80 mm Hg and with the ECG appearance lisinopril was discontinued and amlodipine started along with aspirin. She was admitted for urgent coronary angiography, which identified a critical 99% osteal left anterior descending lesion (Figure 1). The following day she underwent successful coronary artery bypass grafting and made an excellent recovery. Now exactly 2 years later she leads a normal active life, does not smoke, and her blood pressure is 130/70 mm Hg. Her medication is atenolol 100 mg, perindopril 4 mg combined with indapamide 1.5 mg, and aspirin 75 mg daily. She is also taking atorvastatin 20 mg daily and has an LDL-cholesterol consistently below 2.0 mmol/l.[2]

The message

CAD affects women as often as men and no racial group is spared. The symptoms are often atypical and need teasing out. The lipids in this lady were falsely reassuring but lipids are only one part of the cardiovascular risk spectrum and no risk factor should be judged in isolation. An HDL-cholesterol of 2.7 mmol/l in a premenopausal woman would be expected to be protective, especially with an LDL-cholesterol of 2.6 mmol/l and normal triglycerides at 1.0 mmol/l. It is important to treat each patient as an individual and not a statistic and to judge each case in the context of the mode of presentation and overall cardiovascular risk. As far as this patient is concerned, we still need to work on the weight, and the CAMELOT trial suggests that we need to lower her blood pressure further by re-introducing amlodipine.[3]

References

1. Mosca L, Appel LS, Benjamin EJ et al. Evidence-based guidelines for cardiovascular disease prevention in women. Circulation 2004; 109: 672–93.
2. LaRosa JC, Grundy SM, Waters DD et al. Intensive lipid lowering with atorvastatin in patients with stable coronary disease. N Engl J Med 2005; 352: 1425–35.
3. Nissen SE, Tuzcu EM, Libby P et al. Effect of antihypertensive agents on cardiovascular events in patients with coronary disease and normal blood pressure. The CAMELOT Study: a randomised controlled trial. JAMA 2004; 292: 2217–26.

Case 5

CASE STUDY: WOMEN AND CARDIOVASCULAR RISK

James A Underberg

Case study

The case is a 38-year-old woman with a diagnosis of polycystic ovary syndrome (PCOS). She does not smoke, and exercises daily. She is being managed by an endocrinologist and a gynecologist, and currently takes oral contraceptives (demulen), metformin, and aldactone. She is referred for evaluation of cardiovascular risk.

At the time of the visit, her body mass index (BMI) is 36.5 and her waist circumference is 40 inches. Her blood pressure (BP) is 120/70 mm Hg. The remainder of the physical exam is unremarkable.

Lab exam shows a fasting blood sugar of 98 and a recent HbA1c of 5.3%. Lipids show: total cholesterol 228, HDL-cholesterol 90, and LDL-cholesterol (calc) 109; triglycerides 145.

Based on the above findings she does not fulfill the diagnostic criteria for metabolic syndrome, and her Framingham risk score gives her a 10-year coronary heart disease (CHD) risk of < 1%.

She is sent for advanced lipid testing via NMR particle analysis.[1] This shows a significantly elevated LDL particle number of 1814, with an elevated small LDL particle number of 1116. Her LDL particle size, however, is large (pattern A). How can we explain this, and does it affect her cardiovascular risk evaluation and treatment?

Given her low total LDL-cholesterol, and elevated particle number, one would expect her particle size to be small. In the setting of PCOS and presumed insulin resistance this would make sense, perhaps through down-regulation of lipoprotein lipase,[2] and could confer increased cardiovascular risk status.[3] Women with PCOS have also been shown to have elevated levels of hepatic lipase.[4] Her large particle size suggests at least two factors masking this process. Oral contraceptives, estrogen in particular, may serve to down-regulate hepatic lipase, and may account for increased HDL-cholesterol levels.[5] The estrogen will also increase triglyceride synthesis, creating triglyceride-rich VLDL and subsequently LDL particles that

Risk of atherosclerosis	HL activity	LDL-C levels	Pathophysiology of CHD risk
Higher	↑	↑	Elevated concentrations of small, dense LDL
	↓	↑	Increased LDL-C (large, buoyant LDL); impaired reverse cholesterol transport, and, possibly, remnants catabolism
Lower	↓	↓	Impaired reverse cholesterol transport, and, possibly, remnants catabolism
	↑	↓	Increased reverse cholesterol transport, low levels of LDL-C (but small, dense LDL)

Figure 1 Cardiovascular risk, hepatic lipase (HL) activity and LDL-cholesterol (LDL-C) levels. CHD, coronary heart disease. Reproduced from Zambon A et al., Curr Opin Lipidol 2003; 14: 183.

normally would be then hydrolyzed into small dense LDL particles by hepatic lipase. Estrogen alone would probably not inhibit hepatic lipase enough to account for minimal hydrolysis; hence the patient also most likely has a hepatic lipase genetic polymorphism, or deficiency of hepatic lipase.

Hepatic lipase deficiency, in this case perhaps attenuated by PCOS-induced increase in hepatic lipase, is most often caused by a genetic polymorphism in the promoter region (514 C to T) of the hepatic lipase gene (LIPC).[6] The presence of the T allele causes low hepatic lipase activity. Patients with the CT genotype have intermediate activity and those with the CC genotype have the highest levels of hepatic lipase activity. Elevated levels of hepatic lipase are associated with small dense LDL particles (atherogenic dyslipidemia), often also associated with low HDL-cholesterol. The expectation, therefore, would be that presence of the T allele would be cardioprotective. Data in this area, however, have been conflicting. Hepatic lipase also has a ligand-binding function, and is involved in the function of the SRB-1 hepatic scavenger receptor role in reverse cholesterol transport (RCT). Low levels of hepatic lipase may interfere with RCT and affect cardiovascular outcomes adversely. Zambon et al. propose that cardiovascular risk is affected both by hepatic lipase activity levels and LDL-cholesterol levels[6] (see Figure 1).

This particular patient under discussion falls into the category of low LDL-cholesterol and probable low hepatic lipase levels. This would account for her increased levels of large LDL particles, but would also suggest impaired RCT, and increased cardiovascular risk. Regarding treatment for patients with hepatic lipase deficiency, data suggest that patients with the highest hepatic lipase levels and the CC genotype benefit the most from lipid-lowering therapy.[7]

This case is an excellent example of the dyslipidemia that exists in many patients with PCOS. Often these patients are cared for by gynecologists only, and are not evaluated for potential cardiovascular risk soon enough. Her elevated particle number warrants aggressive risk reduction.[8] However, this should be managed within the context of her plans for pregnancy. Weight loss and management of her insulin resistance are important. Her hepatic lipase abnormality and oral contraceptive therapy might fool the practitioner into underestimating her risk, given her elevated HDL-cholesterol and large LDL particle size. Starting the patient on a bile acid sequestrate (pregnancy category B) would be useful, with close monitoring of her triglycerides status. This would lower her LDL particle number.[9] If she was not considering pregnancy, low-dose statin therapy with a hydrophilic statin such as pravastatin or rosuvastatin might be appropriate, with a goal of bringing her LDL particle number down below 1000,[10] and with the understanding that her benefit might be less than in those with elevated hepatic lipase levels.

References

1. Otvos J. Measurement of triglyceride rich lipoproteins by nuclear magnetic resonance spectroscopy. Clin Cardiol 1999; 22 (Suppl 6): II21–II27.
2. Ginsberg H. Insulin resistance and cardiovascular disease. J Clin Invest 2000; 106: 453–8.
3. Benlian P, De Gennes JL. Foubert L et al. Premature atherosclerosis in patients with familial chylomicronemia caused by mutations in the lipoprotein lipase gene. N Engl J Med 1996; 335: 848–54.
4. Pirwany IR, Fleming R, Greer IA, Packard CJ, Sattar N. Lipids and lipoprotein subfractions in women with PCOS: relationship to metabolic and endocrine parameters. Clin Endocrinol 2001; 54: 447–53.
5. Schaefer EJ, Foster DM, Zech LA, et al. The effects of estrogen administration on plasma lipoprotein metabolism in premenopausal females. J Clin Endocrinol Metab, 1983; 57: 262–7.
6. Zambon A, Deeb SS, Pauletto P, Crepaldi G, Brunzell JD. Hepatic lipase: a marker for cardiovascular disease risk and response to therapy. Curr Opin Lipidol 2003; 14: 179–89.

7. Zambon A, Deeb SS, Brown BG et al. A common hepatic lipase gene promoter variant determines clinical response to intensive lipid-lowering treatment. Circulation 2001; 103: 792–8.
8. Cromwell WC, Otvos JD. Low density lipoprotein particle number and risk for cardiovascular disease. Curr Atheroscler Rep 2004; 6: 381–7.
9. Rosenson R. Colesevelam HCL reduces LDL particle number and increases LDL size in hypercholesterolemia. Atherosclerosis 2006; 185: 327–30.
10. Underberg JA. Use of statins in women of child bearing age. Lipid Spin 2006; 3: 6–8.

Case 6

A PATIENT WITH DIABETES AND CORONARY HEART DISEASE

Mikko Syvänne

Case study

I was about to start my cardiology evening practice one day in June, 1999, when a worried colleague asked if I could fit in an extra patient on whom he had just performed an exercise test. 'I'm unsure about the interpretation,' he said. 'I didn't dare to exercise him further because his blood pressure rose so ominously.'

I encountered a previously healthy 54-year-old man. I learned that he was an architect and an amateur musician, his family presenting world class talent in classical music. I will call him Pekka (a common Finnish man's name, not his real one).

Pekka had contacted a general practitioner a few days earlier. According to the colleague's notes Pekka had been stressed and nervous, and 3 days earlier he had experienced shortness of breath and vague chest compression. He was tachycardic at 90 beats per minute (bpm) and his blood pressure was 180/110 mm Hg. An electrocardiogram was unremarkable. He was prescribed low doses of oxazepam and propranolol and referred for an exercise test.

Further medical history revealed that Pekka had been experiencing rather typical anginal chest discomfort for a week or so. Although he had been asymptomatic at rest, his angina was severe and new-onset; therefore, it was unstable, type IB according to Braunwald's classification. He had no family history of coronary heart disease (CHD). He had never smoked. There was no previous history of hypertension, hyperlipidemia or diabetes, although none of these had been evaluated lately. He was abdominally obese, 182 cm, 112 kg, with a body mass index (BMI) of 34 kg/m^2. Otherwise physical examination was unremarkable.

The bicycle ergometry exercise test had been terminated early at 100 watts and heart rate 116 bpm as blood pressure rose from 162/108 to 265/135 mm Hg. Pekka recalled some chest discomfort after termination of the test. At peak exercise there was a down-sloping ST segment depression of 2.3 mm in lead V6 and somewhat milder in V5. Although there was voltage evidence of left ventricular hypertrophy, reducing the specificity of the ECG finding, little doubt remained that Pekka had significant coronary artery disease.

The Bayesian pre-test likelihood of coronary disease hit the ceiling when risk factor assessment was completed: fasting blood glucose was 11.0 mmol/l, cholesterol 6.8, HDL-cholesterol 1.3, triglycerides 2.31 and LDL-cholesterol 4.5 mmol/l.

A few days later coronary angiography showed a tight stenosis in the mid left anterior descending (LAD) artery (Figure 1A). The circumflex branch and the right coronary artery had nonsignificant luminal irregularities. Nonsignificant? Yes, in the sense that they were not severe enough to cause myocardial ischemia or symptoms. But, on the other hand, highly significant in the sense that they certainly contained abundant soft, vulnerable plaque, prone to rupture and cause unstable angina, myocardial infarction or sudden death. As I'm writing this 6 years after the angiogram was obtained, Pekka remains alive, free of coronary events and symptoms.

The LAD was immediately stented (Figure 1). Pekka was discharged on bisoprolol 5 mg bid, aspirin 100 mg, clopidogrel for the next 4 weeks, and simvastatin 20 mg daily.

According to a paper by Haffner et al., published in the previous year,[1] in a Finnish population, followed up for 7 years, those with diabetes and established CHD had a cardiovascular mortality of 42%, contrasted with about 15% in diabetic people without coronary disease as well as people without diabetes but with coronary disease, and only 2% in those with neither of these conditions. Therefore, it was quite clear from the outset that secondary prevention was to play a paramount role in Pekka's management. As mentioned, he was immediately put on aspirin and a statin. A selective beta-blocker was a natural initial choice for blood pressure control, as it would also help to control any residual or recurrent ischemia and might be life-saving in case of a future acute event. In 1999 all these approaches had already been proven to be at least as useful in people with diabetes as in others, and equally safe.

Clearly, lifestyle intervention was literally at the heart of the matter. Pekka quite enthusiastically adopted qualitative dietary changes to reduce saturated fat and simple carbohydrates, making exciting culinary discoveries in the realm of fish and vegetables. Although his favorite past-time activities centered on music rather than exercise, he did get a fair amount of the latter by regularly walking a part of his daily commuter travel. Weight control was harder. Pekka did not like weighing himself, and at first no progress was made. I did not resort to weight-losing pharmacotherapy, finding the available options cumbersome, of limited value, and lacking evidence in hard endpoints. This may change if the endocannabinoid receptor blockers hold their promise.

The point, I think, is that much can be achieved in prevention even if weight loss fails. It would be unethical to deny evidence-based preventive measures from

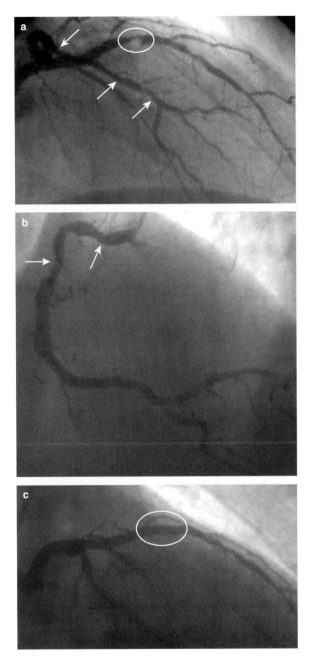

Figure 1 (a) A critical stenosis in the left anterior descending (LAD) branch of the left coronary artery (ellipse) and lesser stenoses in the circumflex branch (arrows). (b) Luminal irregularities in the right coronary artery. (c) LAD after stent deployment (ellipse).

25

people unable to lose weight. Of course, targets become easier to achieve if weight control is successful.

Much work remained to be done. One month after the angioplasty Pekka was feeling fine. His blood pressure was 200/100 mm Hg on bisoprolol. I decided to focus on this first. Even with a highly cooperative person with an academic background, such as Pekka, there are limits in the adoption of new things. There was also the understandable shock of newly diagnosed disease with a reluctance to 'take too many pills.' I knew there were many more pills to come, but I kept it to myself at this point. I changed the beta-blocker to a combination pill with the same dose of bisoprolol plus a low dose of thiazide and added a calcium channel blocker, amlodipine, starting at 5 mg.

Physicians sometimes find comprehensive risk factor control formidably complex and time-consuming. 'I only have 15 minutes, how can I fix somebody's lifestyle, lipids, glycemia and blood pressure in that time?'. You can't, and you don't need to. You can, and you should, go stepwise. Rome wasn't built in a day.

About 4 months after the angioplasty Pekka continued to be asymptomatic, so the risk of significant in-stent restenosis was almost over. Blood pressure varied around 140/85 mm Hg. Cholesterol was 3.9, HDL-cholesterol 1.2, triglycerides 1.67, and LDL-cholesterol 2.0 mmol/l, so we were well in the target range. Fasting blood glucose was somewhat improved at 9.3 mmol/l.

During the following year, blood pressure control was borderline at about 150–160/75–90 mm Hg. Increasing amlodipine to 10 mg almost fixed this but, prompted by the then-published Heart Outcomes Prevention Evaluation (HOPE) trial, the ACE inhibitor ramipril was added and gradually titrated up to 10 mg.

Eventually, by the end of 2002, a gradual weight loss of about 10 kg had taken place in spite of the initial difficulties. This was clearly reflected in the lipid values: with the same simvastatin 20 mg regimen total cholesterol was down to 3.4, HDL-cholesterol 1.3, triglycerides 1.25 and LDL-cholesterol 1.5 mmol/l. Thus, ahead of time, we had reached the targets later suggested by studies such as the Heart Protection Study (HPS), the Pravastatin or Atorvastatin Evaluation and Infection Trial (PROVE IT) and the Treating to New Targets (TNT).

I see diabetologists frowning at my negligence in glycemic control in a diabetic person. In fact, fasting blood glucose remained steadily high at 9 mmol/l and HbA1c ranged from 6.1 to 6.5% (upper limit of normal, 6.0%). In addition to the psychological barriers referred to above, I gave glycemia the lowest priority because of the modest cardiovascular benefit seen in the UK Prospective Diabetes Study (UKPDS) trial.[2] However, 2 years after the angioplasty, when lifestyle measures had no further effect, I started metformin, gradually titrating the dose up to 2 g per day. Fasting blood sugar fell down to 7.6 mmol/l and HbA1c to 6.0 mmol/l. Recently I referred Pekka to a diabetologist for consideration to participate in a randomized trial comparing intensive glycemic control with glargine insulin to standard care.

Among others, the Steno-2 trial[3] has shown that comprehensive intensive risk factor management in high-risk people with diabetes yields major benefits in cardiovascular prevention. The current LDL-cholesterol target in a high-risk diabetic patient such as Pekka is well below 2 mmol/l. This was easily achieved with lifestyle intervention and 20 mg simvastatin, as it is in most (although not all) patients. Yet, surveys such as EUROASPIRE 2 show that this easy, safe, and nowadays relatively inexpensive therapy is neglected in a distressingly high proportion of those who would benefit.

References

1. Haffner SM, Lehto S, Rönnemaa T, Pyörälä K, Laakso M. Mortality from coronary heart disease in subjects with type 2 diabetes and in nondiabetic subjects with and without prior myocardial infarction. N Engl J Med 1998; 339: 229–32.
2. UK Prospective Diabetes Study (UKPDS) Group. Intensive blood-glucose control with sulphonylureas or insulin compared with conventional treatment and risk of complications in patients with type 2 diabetes (UKPDS 33). Lancet 1998; 352: 837–53.
3. Gæde P, Vedel P, Larsen N, Jensen GVH, et al. Multifactorial intervention and cardiovascular disease in patients with type 2 diabetes. N Engl J Med 2003; 348: 383–93.

Case 7

LIPID–MODIFYING THERAPY IN A PERSON WITH DIABETES AND AN ACUTE CORONARY SYNDROME

Andrew M Tonkin and Lei Chen

Case study

A 68-year-old man presents to the emergency department at 9 pm after experiencing nausea and shortness of breath since 1 pm that day. He has no history of chest discomfort but has noticed increasing exertional dyspnea for 6 months.

He is known to have diabetes, treated with an oral hypoglycemic agent. He has a 30 pack-year history of smoking before stopping 6 years before. He has lived alone since his wife died 2 years previously.

His pulse is 96 bpm and regular. Blood pressure is 152/88 mm Hg. An ECG shows 1.5 mm ST depression in leads V2–V4. There are no hospital beds available and it is decided to keep him in the emergency department. He is commenced on aspirin, heparin, and a beta-blocker while troponin I level is awaited. This is initially borderline (0.5 mg/ml, with laboratory upper limit of normal 0.4 mg/ml). The next morning his ECG shows anteroseptal T wave inversion and repeat troponin I level is 2.2 mg/ml. His fasting lipid levels show total cholesterol 5.6 mmol/l, HDL-cholesterol 0.8 mmol/l, and triglycerides 2.4 mmol/l. A provisional laboratory diagnosis of nonST segment elevation myocardial infarction is made. He is admitted to the Coronary Care Unit (CCU) and commenced on intravenous nitroglycerin.

In the CCU, a statin and an ACE inhibitor are also commenced. Because of the patient's age, history of diabetes, and elevated troponin I level, he is assessed as being at high risk and coronary angiography is recommended. This shows an 80% stenosis in the proximal left anterior descending (LAD) coronary artery with angiographic appearances consistent with thrombus formation. There are nonflow-limiting stenoses in the circumflex or right coronary artery. The left ventriculogram shows anterior hypokinesis. A drug-eluting stent is deployed successfully to the lesion in the LAD coronary artery.

Discussion

The evidence base for the efficacy of lipid-modifying therapy in prevention of recurrent cardiovascular events in patients with coronary heart disease (CHD) is overwhelming. Initial landmark trials of statins including 4S, CARE, and LIPID enrolled patients some time after an acute coronary syndrome. The Heart Protection Study[1] extended these observations in showing that future events could also be prevented in those with low baseline LDL-cholesterol levels (as low as 3.5 mmol/l). Both the Heart Protection Study[1] and CARDS showed the benefits of statins in people with diabetes.

Measurement of fasting lipids including HDL-cholesterol and triglycerides as well as LDL-cholesterol should be done as a routine in all patients admitted with CHD events. More than 24 hours after admission with acute coronary syndromes, hormone changes modify levels and reliable estimates can only be obtained after about a further 6 weeks.

In the initial landmark trials, recruitment was delayed after any acute coronary syndrome, as it was thought that statins would not impact on the processes associated with coronary plaque instability and left ventricular remodelling. During the earliest 2–3 months after an acute coronary syndrome, there is an increased risk of future events including myocardial infarction and death compared with patients with stable CHD. However, studies such as CHAMP and register studies did show benefit if statins were commenced before discharge. Concordance is increased with in-hospital initiation close to the index event.

The most robust data for statins after acute coronary syndromes are provided by those trials in which randomization occurred very early. These trials particularly included PROVE-IT TIMI 22[2] and A to Z.[3] PROVE-IT TIMI 22[2] compared 40 mg pravastatin daily and 80 mg atorvastatin daily in 4162 patients randomized at a mean of 7 days after an acute coronary syndrome. Median LDL-cholesterol achieved during treatment was 2.46 mmol/l and 1.60 mmol/l, respectively ($p < 0.001$). Over a mean 24 months follow-up, the primary endpoint, a composite of all-cause death, myocardial infarction, unstable angina requiring rehospitalization, revascularization, and stroke was reduced from 26.3% in the pravastatin group to 22.4% in the atorvastatin group ($p = 0.005$). The A to Z trial[3] compared early initiation of an intensive statin regimen (40 mg daily of simvastatin for 1 month then 80 mg simvastatin daily) with delayed initiation of a less intensive regimen (placebo for 4 months then 20 mg simvastatin daily) in 4497 patients following the acute coronary syndrome. Mean LDL-cholesterol at 8 months was 1.63 mmol/l and 1.99 mmol/l, respectively. The primary endpoint, a composite of cardiovascular death, nonfatal myocardial infarction, readmission for an acute coronary syndrome and stroke occurred in 16.7% of the less intensively treated group and 14.4% in the more intensively treated group over 24 months

30

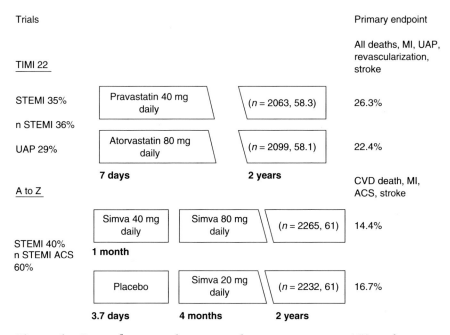

Figure 1 Design features and primary endpoints in recent post-ACS trials. STEMI, ST segment elevation myocardial infarction; n STEMI, nonST segment elevation myocardial infarction; ACS, acute coronary syndromes; MI, myocardial infarction; UAP, unstable angina pectoris; CVD, cardiovascular disease; simva, simvastatin. Values in brackets are expressed as number and average age of the participants.

($p=0.14$). Cardiovascular death was reduced with more intensive therapy (4.1% vs 5.4%, $p=0.05$). These results are not inconsistent with PROVE-IT TIMI 22. Results are summarized in Figure 1.

What LDL-cholesterol level should be targeted? Further evidence concerning this is obtained from the TNT study in stable CHD patients. After an 8 week period of open-label treatment with atorvastatin 10 mg daily, 1001 subjects who had LDL-cholesterol level < 3.4 mmol/l were randomized to either atorvastatin 10 mg or 80 mg daily and followed for a median of 4.9 years. The primary endpoint, a composite of CHD death, nonfatal nonprocedural-related myocardial infarction, resuscitation after cardiac arrest or fatal or nonfatal stroke occurred in 10.9% of subjects given 10 mg atorvastatin daily (who achieved a mean LDL-cholesterol of 2.6 mmol/l) and 8.7% of those given 80 mg atorvastatin daily (mean LDL-cholesterol level 2.0 mmol/l) ($p < 0.001$). In the light of these trials, among other authorities, the Adult Treatment Panel III of the US National Cholesterol Education Program concluded in a published update that an

LDL-cholesterol target of 1.8 mmol/l (70 mg/dl) was a very reasonable therapeutic option in patients at very high risk of future events, such as those with known CHD.

Considerations of potential benefit:risk balance are relevant with all therapies. Although an overview of the data shows a relationship between doses of statins and side effects, major toxicity is uncommon. Using more intensive therapy with higher doses of statins, approximately one major vascular event is prevented with a treatment of approximately 40 patients over 2 years. This far outweighs adverse effects, particularly when factors that might increase the risk of side effects are taken into account.

Current guidelines focus on LDL-cholesterol targets and, to a lesser extent, HDL-cholesterol and nonHDL-cholesterol in those with elevated triglyceride levels. This may change in the future. Further analyses of PROVE-IT TIMI 22 have shown that vascular events were most decreased when LDL-cholesterol was reduced to < 1.8 mmol/l and CRP to < 2 mg/l. Future guidelines may also include apolipoprotein B as a therapeutic target, particularly in people with diabetes such as the patient described. The evidence is increasing to suggest that this measure of LDL particle number is superior to LDL concentration in its predictive ability. The measurement of LDL particle number via apolipoprotein B levels is particularly relevant when there is an increase in more atherogenic small, dense rather than large buoyant LDL particles. Small dense particles are the predominant phenotype in those with triglyceride levels > 1.8 mmol/l.

In summary, people with diabetes often have atypical symptoms associated with coronary atherosclerosis such as in this patient or indeed more often have 'silent' ischemia. The presence of diabetes increases both case-fatality rates with acute coronary syndromes and subsequent long-term prognosis.

The patient was categorized as being at high risk after his nonST elevation myocardial infarction, and was treated appropriately with an early invasive strategy with angiography and subsequent stent deployment. It is still unclear as to the extent to which drug-eluting stents will improve long-term outcomes in people with diabetes. Although he had no other major coronary stenoses at angiography, almost certainly he has diffuse coronary atherosclerosis. On the background of lifestyle therapy he requires an aggressive approach to LDL-cholesterol-lowering with a statin, with an LDL-cholesterol target suggested by recent trials to be around 1.8 mmol/l.

Pending further data from ongoing studies in people with diabetes, a case could be made for combined therapy with a statin and micronized fenofibrate, particularly if the patient has features of typical dyslipidemia associated with diabetes, including low HDL-cholesterol and elevated triglycerides. Analyses of the VA-HIT study showed particular benefit of gemfibrozil in CHD patients with such features of the metabolic syndrome. This benefit was seen without reduction in LDL-cholesterol. Also, the risk associated with low HDL-cholesterol persists in CHD patients even when they are treated with a statin. However, patients should be monitored for possible creatine phosphokinase elevation on such combined therapy, although fenofibrate does not share the same pharmacokinetic interaction of gemfibrozil with statins, nor other statins the relatively high incidence of rhabdomyolysis seen with cerivastatin.

References

1. Heart Protection Study Collaborative Group. MRC/BHF Heart Protection Study of cholesterol lowering with simvastatin in 20,536 high-risk individuals: a randomised placebo-controlled trial. Lancet 2002; 360: 7–22.
2. Cannon CP, Braunwald E, McCabe CH et al. Intensive versus moderate lipid lowering with statins after acute coronary syndromes. N Engl J Med 2004; 350: 1495–504.
3. de Lemos JA, Blazing MA, Wiviott SD et al. Early intensive vs a delayed conservative simvastatin strategy in patients with acute coronary syndromes: phase Z of the A to Z trial. JAMA 2004; 292: 1307–16.

Case 8

A PATIENT WITH THE CLINICAL PHENOTYPE OF SEVERE FAMILIAL HYPERCHOLESTEROLEMIA

Anton FH Stalenhoef

Familial hypercholesterolemia

Familial hypercholesterolemia (FH) is an autosomal dominant inherited lipid disorder caused by one of the many mutations in the gene for the LDL receptor, leading to increased total cholesterol and LDL-cholesterol levels (two times elevated), typical tendon xanthomata, and premature atherosclerosis. The clinical expression varies widely and is influenced by other risk factors. The disorder occurs in 1 in 400–500 individuals; in certain areas in the world, the incidence is much higher due to a founder effect. Homozygous patients with two mutated LDL receptor alleles (total serum cholesterol four times elevated) develop xanthomata and atherosclerosis at a young age. If untreated they usually die before the age of 20–30 years due to complications of vascular disease. The FH clinical phenotype can also result from mutations in the gene for apolipoprotein B, the ligand of LDL for the LDL receptor. In addition to common mutations in the LDL receptor and apolipoprotein B genes, two rare mutations in genes involved in cholesterol metabolism have recently been described to cause severe hypercholesterolemia. The following case is a typical example of a patient with a severe clinical FH phenotype.

Description of the case

The patient JV (female, 19 years old, born in 1983) was diagnosed early in 2002 with FH on the basis of severely elevated total serum cholesterol concentration (16 mmol/l) and the presence of Achilles tendon xanthomata and corneal arcus. She was treated with a high dose of atorvastatin and cholestyramine 4 g/day. Because her serum cholesterol level remained above 10 mmol/l, she was referred in February 2003 to our University Medical Centre for further treatment. At that

35

time she did not have symptoms of angina or other cardiovascular complaints, except for some fatigue. She never smoked. She worked as an obstetric nurse. In addition to the above-mentioned medication she had used an oral contraceptive agent for 2 years. Her father was also known to have elevated serum cholesterol (10 mmol/l), for which he received drug treatment. His brother had died at the age of 36 years from an acute coronary event. This brother's serum cholesterol was not known, but several other siblings of the father had elevated serum cholesterol. JV's mother had a normal total serum cholesterol level of 4.9 mmol/l. JV did not have siblings.

On physical examination JV was slightly overweight (height 1.71 m, body weight 75.7 kg, BMI 25.9 kg/m^2), waist circumference 80 cm, blood pressure 120/70 mm Hg, pulse rate 72/min. She exhibited inferior corneal arcus in both eyes and clearly thickened Achilles tendons. There were otherwise no abnormalities on physical examination.

Laboratory investigation at the first visit in our clinic revealed a total serum cholesterol on treatment of 11.4 mmol/l, LDL-cholesterol 10.1 mmol/l, triglycerides 0.89 mmol/l, HDL-cholesterol 0.98 mmol/l, and the Lp(a) concentration was 806 mg/l (N < 300 mg/dl). Glucose was 4.0 mmol/l, thyroid function was normal, and there was no microalbuminuria. Additional blood chemistry tests were normal. Her ECG showed a sinus rhythm without clear abnormalities, in particular there were no signs of ischemia or previous infarctions. Thus, we confirmed the clinical diagnosis of classical severe familial hypercholesterolemia, apparently heterozygous form, because her mother was normocholesterolemic. The patient's DNA was analyzed for mutations in the LDL receptor and apolipoprotein B genes, but surprisingly, no mutations after sequencing in both these genes could be demonstrated (Dr J. Defesche, AMC, Amsterdam). In rare cases, the FH clinical phenotype can also result from mutations in the gene proprotein convertase subtilisin/kexin type 9 (PCSK9) encoding for neural apoptosis-regulated convertase 1 (NARC-1) and in the autosomal recessive hypercholesterolemia (ARH) gene, which encodes an adaptor protein which is necessary for LDL endocytosis.[1] Analysis of these mutations has not been performed yet, although the latter recessive form seems less likely because the father had clear hypercholesterolemia.

Clinical course

Because of the presence of severely elevated plasma LDL-cholesterol levels and corneal arcus at a young age, as is observed in patients with homozygous FH, bi-weekly treatment with LDL apheresis was considered. However, because of the rather heavy burden for the patient and the high cost of this treatment, combined

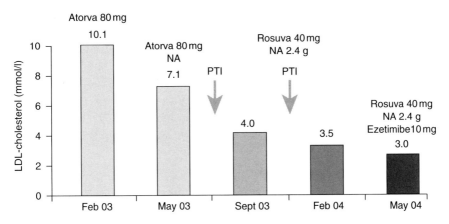

Figure 1 *LDL-cholesterol levels during pharmacological treatment. Atorva,*
atorvastatin; NA, nicotinic acid; Rosuva, rosuvastatin; PTI, percutaneous
transluminal intervention.

drug therapy was instituted first to see what level of LDL-cholesterol could be
obtained. The combination of atorvastatin 80 mg/day, later rosuvastatin
40 mg/day, increasing doses of nicotinic acid up to three times 0.8 g/day, and
ezetimibe 10 mg/day resulted in a gradual decrease of LDL-cholesterol to a
sustained level of around 3.0 mmol/l (Figure 1). Unfortunately, after 7–8 months
the patient experienced periods of angina for which she had to be hospitalized
twice. She underwent coronary interventions (dotter and stenting procedures). A
distal occlusion in the left anterior descending (LAD) branch was not accessible
for percutaneous coronary intervention or bypass surgery. After these procedures
echocardiography revealed a normal left ventricular function and also exercise
testing did not show clear abnormalities. Medical treatment was expanded with
beta-blockers, aspirin, and clopidogrel, while the oral contraceptive was stopped.
The medication was tolerated well and laboratory safety tests remained normal.
After the last procedure in November 2004, the patient no longer had chest
complaints (last clinic visit summer 2005) and could restart her work as an
obstetric assistant again.

Evaluation

The clinical presentation of this young woman with severe familial
hypercholesterolemia and early onset of coronary disease resembles the clinical
course of a patient with the homozygous form of FH. The molecular genetic
defect in this patient is not known, because DNA analysis of the LDL receptor and

apolipoprotein B genes revealed no mutations. In addition, her mother was normocholesterolemic, excluding classical homozygous FH. Whatever the molecular defect that may have caused the severe hypercholesterolemia in this patient, she was responsive to intensive pharmacological treatment. Combination therapy with high doses of potent statins, nicotinic acid, and the cholesterol absorption inhibitor ezetimibe eventually reduced her LDL-cholesterol more than 75% to a remarkable level of around 3.0 mmol/l, which averted the necessity to perform LDL apheresis. Unfortunately for the patient, this treatment was instituted too late to prevent coronary disease. When to begin treatment in children with familial hypercholesterolemia and to what extent has been a matter of debate. Statin treatment of FH children (mean age 13 years) for 2 years appears to be safe and is associated with an attenuation of progression of the carotid intima media thickness.[2] Clearly, if the diagnosis in this patient had been made earlier, she would have been eligible for intensive treatment at a young age on the basis of her LDL level and family history, irrespective of the molecular defect. Regarding possible future wishes with respect to pregnancy and the necessity to interrupt pharmacological therapy in this patient, temporary treatment with LDL apheresis would be a therapeutic option,[3] although the long-term prognosis regarding life expectancy seems less favorable in this patient.

References

1. Rader DJ, Cohen J, Hobbs HH. Monogenetic hypercholesterolemia: new insights in pathogenesis and treatment. J Clin Invest 2003; 111: 1795–803.
2. Wiegman A, Hutten BA, de Groot E et al. Efficacy and safety of statin therapy in children with familial hypercholesterolemia: a randomized controlled trial. JAMA 2004; 292: 331–7.
3. Kroon AA, Swinkels DW, van Dongen PW, Stalenhoef AF. Pregnancy in a patient with homozygous familial hypercholesterolemia treated with long-term low-density lipoprotein apheresis. Metabolism 1994; 43: 1164–70.

Case 9

A Case Of Successful Treatment Of Familial Hypercholesterolemia

Anders G Olsson

Case study

The patient is a 49-year-old man in a family with known hypercholesterolemia (FH). His father died of myocardial infarction at age 40, and his brother has FH.

His FH was detected in 1976 at age 20 (Table 1). At physical examination corneal arcus were noted and he also showed small tendinous xanthomata on extensor tendons of digits 2 to 4 bilaterally. Physical status was otherwise normal, as well as systolic and diastolic blood pressure. He was also a smoker but stopped at age 32. He is a married controller. He maintains a strict hypocholesterolemic diet and exercises regularly.

At the age of 20 the patient was already being treated with a combination of cholestyramine 12 g daily and nicotinic acid 6 g daily, with limited effect on serum cholesterol. In spite of this treatment total cholesterol was 11.1 mmol/l (Table 1). The patient found the treatment unpleasant and complained of side effects. When simvastatin became available in 1985 he was therefore immediately treated with it at a dose of 20 mg and then 40 mg daily plus cholestyramine 8–16 g daily. Initially there was a reasonably good effect with the combination of 40 mg simvastatin plus 8 g of cholestyramine but after some years of treatment a successive escape of the effect on LDL-cholesterol was noted (Table 1). Simvastatin dose was increased to 80 mg daily. Plasma exchange at 10-day intervals was therefore started, later changed to specific LDL apheresis. Atorvastatin 80 mg and later 120 mg daily was substituted for simvastatin. With this regimen total cholesterol and LDL-cholesterol before apheresis were 6.2 and 4.4 mmol/l, respectively. Figure 1 demonstrates the effect of the addition of ezetimibe to the treatment with atorvastatin and apheresis. Rosuvastatin 80 mg daily was then substituted for atorvastatin. On the combination of rosuvastatin and ezetimibe total cholesterol and LDL-cholesterol decreased to 3.8 and 2.2 mmol/l, respectively, and have subsequently been maintained at 4.3 and 2.4 mmol/l, with HDL-cholesterol about 1.3 mmol/l and triglycerides about 0.8 mmol/l. The combination treatment has helped the patient to reach his LDL-cholesterol target. Apheresis was thereby made redundant and was stopped.

Table 1 Total cholesterol and LDL-cholesterol (mmol/l) levels before and during various treatments

Cholesterol	At detection	Nic + Q	S20	S40	S40 + Q early	S40 + Q late	A120	R80 + E10
Total	12.4	11.1	8.6	6.6	5.8	7.9	6.2	3.8
LDL	10.9	9.0	7.4	5.2	4.3	6.5	4.4	2.2

Nic, nicotinic acid 6 g; Q, cholestyramine 8–16 g; S20 and S40, simvastatin 20 and 40 mg; A120, atorvastatin 120 mg before apheresis; R80, rosuvastatin 80 mg; E10, ezetimibe 10 mg; all daily doses.

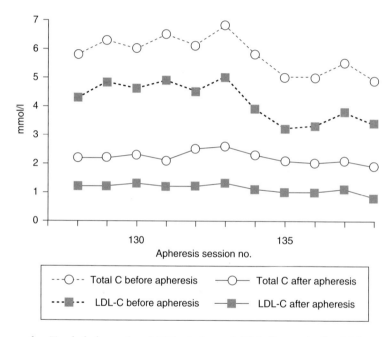

Figure 1 *Total cholesterol and LDL-cholesterol (C) before and after LDL apheresis. The apheresis interval was 10 days. Drug treatment was atorvastatin 120 mg daily during the whole period. Ezetimibe 10 mg daily was given after apheresis session no. 133.*

Liver transaminases have been at the upper limit of normal for both s-ASAT and s-ALAT. The patient has complained of back pain and now and then some weak muscular pain. CK has always stayed normal.

Today the patient is completely free of ischemic symptoms. A determination of intima-media thickness of the carotid arteries at age 49 showed only slight increases without atherosclerotic plaques.

40

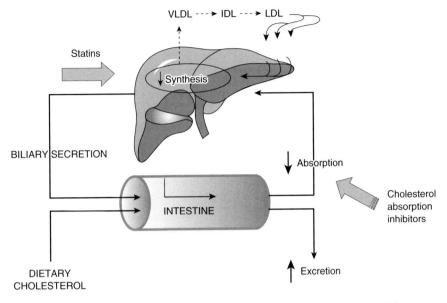

Figure 2 Site of action of statins and selective cholesterol absorption inhibitors.

Comment

The case illustrates the tremendous change in hypolipidemic treatment that has occurred during the last 20 years. It also shows how treatment goals with the availability of ever-increasing lipid-lowering potency of the drug have been pushed down. Then a combination of high doses of the most efficient lipid-lowering drugs available hardly influenced the serum cholesterol concentration, but nevertheless induced quite marked subjective side effects. Now the combination of a high dose of the most efficient statin on the market with a cholesterol absorption inhibitor can move total and LDL cholesterol levels in markedly hypercholesterolemic FH patients from extreme levels to below the average of the normal population, and this without subjective side effects.

The cholesterol absorption inhibitor is a valuable new tool to bring down high LDL-cholesterol levels in severely affected individuals, such as those with FH.[1] This is also the case in patients with coronary heart disease[2] and in patients with diabetes mellitus and the metabolic syndrome.[3] Statin and cholesterol absorption inhibitors act at different levels in the cholesterol metabolism and therefore an additive effect is achieved by the combined treatment (Figure 2). The role of cholesterol synthesis and absorption and the importance of these functions in cholesterol homeostasis have been extensively studied by Miettinen et al.[4] Blood LDL-cholesterol levels are highly dependent on the cholesterol synthetic rate, mainly in the liver, and of cholesterol absorption from the intestine. Miettinen's group of researchers has developed methods to estimate cholesterol synthesis and absorption by determining certain tracers in blood. In particular, a high serum cholestanol/cholesterol ratio indicates a high absorption and low synthesis of cholesterol. This subgroup did not benefit very much from simvastatin treatment in the 4S trial. This is understandable since statins exert their effect by inhibiting cholesterol synthesis.

In the present case, presenting with typical FH, we could primarily assume a high cholesterol synthesis because of the partial lack of LDL receptors on the liver cells and the subsequent feedback on cholesterol synthesis. Consequently we also noted a substantial but limited effect of statin treatment on LDL-cholesterol concentrations in blood. However, the patient responded equally well to the addition of the cholesterol absorption inhibitor ezetimibe, indicating that he was also a high cholesterol absorber. His almost complete lack of signs of increasing atherosclerosis at age 50 contrasts with his father's death from acute myocardial infarction at age 40. It is highly likely that the patient's healthy arteries at this age are due to a successful lifestyle and drug treatment.

References

1. Stein E, Stender S, Mata P et al. Achieving lipoprotein goals in patients at high risk with severe hypercholesterolemia: efficacy and safety of ezetimibe co-administered with atorvastatin. American Heart Journal 2004; 148: 447–55.
2. Brohet C, Banai S, Alings A et al. LDL-C goal attainment with the addition of ezetimibe to ongoing simvastatin treatment in coronary heart disease patients with hypercholesterolemia. Curr Med Res Opin 2005; 21: 571–8.
3. Simons L, Tonkon M, Masana L et al. Effects of ezetimibe added to on-going statin therapy on the lipid profile of hypercholesterolemic patients with diabetes mellitus or metabolic syndrome. Curr Med Res Opin 2004; 20: 1437–45.
4. Miettinen TA, Strandberg TE, Gylling H. Noncholesterol sterols and cholesterol lowering by long-term simvastatin treatment in coronary patients: relation to basal serum cholestanol. Arterioscler Thromb Vasc Biol 2000; 20: 1340–6.

Case 10

LDL Apheresis Therapy During Pregnancy

Linda C Hemphill

Case study

Patient CB, a 39-year-old female, presented in October 1997 with out of hospital cardiac arrest. She had no previous history of coronary artery disease. Her husband instituted cardiopulmonary resuscitation and she was transported to a local hospital where acute inferior myocardial infarction (MI) was diagnosed. Positive low-level exercise stress test post MI led to coronary angiography, which showed high grade left main stenosis, diffuse mild disease in the mid left anterior descending and diffuse moderate disease in the proximal and mid circumflex. The right coronary artery was totally occluded. She subsequently underwent four-vessel coronary artery bypass graft surgery in November 1997.

Admission blood work revealed an elevated total cholesterol of 9.07 mmol/l. She was treated with HMG-CoA reductase inhibitor therapy ('statin' therapy) through 1998 and early 1999 and remained asymptomatic with regard to her coronary artery disease. In February 1999, the patient became pregnant and immediately stopped statin therapy. Attempts to lower her cholesterol with diet and a bile acid sequestrant were inadequate. In May 1999 her total cholesterol was 8.50 mmol/l and LDL-cholesterol 5.96 mmol/l on 30 g of colestipol, a regimen she was finding difficult to maintain. She was referred for heparin-induced extracorporeal LDL precipitation (HELP) apheresis therapy.

In June 1999, bi-weekly HELP treatments were begun and continued through the 38th week of pregnancy for a total of eight treatments. Treatment sessions were uneventful. Vital signs were stable and she remained asymptomatic. The selective removal of apo B-containing lipoproteins with LDL apheresis causes sawtooth-like alterations in lipoprotein concentrations (Figure 1). Prior to treatments, her mean total cholesterol was 9.87 mmol/l and LDL-cholesterol was 7.05 mmol/l. Post treatment means were 6.40 mmol/l and 4.12 mmol/l, respectively.

Fetal assessment was determined by serial fetal ultrasound and weekly nonstress tests after 32 weeks, all of which were normal. Nonstress test was also performed during her third HELP treatment and was reactive (normal). Induction

43

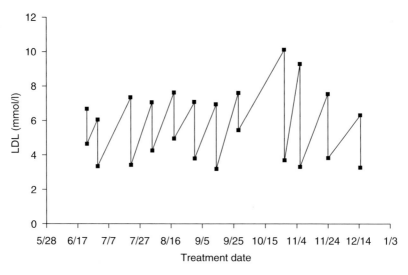

Figure 1 LDL apheresis in a pregnant patient.

of labor was performed on October 6, at 39 weeks. She had a spontaneous vaginal delivery of a girl weighing 3095 g with Apgars of 9/9.

She resumed HELP therapy after a 1 month hiatus and continued for 2 months post delivery in order to remain off statin therapy while breast-feeding. Her first pre-apheresis LDL after this hiatus was 10.10 mmol/l – her baseline off all therapy, including sequestrant. Her pre-apheresis LDLs during this period show the well described decline over time seen when apheresis is instituted and which, generally reach a steady state by 3–6 months of apheresis therapy (Figure 1). Before these treatments, her mean total cholesterol was 10.23 mmol/l and LDL-cholesterol was 8.32 mmol/l. Post treatment means were 5.13 mmol/l and 3.52 mmol/l, respectively.

Comments

Pregnancy in patients with severe hypercholesterolemia and coronary artery disease presents multiple problems for both mother and fetus. The most potent agents for LDL-cholesterol reduction, the HMG-CoA reductase inhibitors ('statins'), must be withheld during pregnancy. Furthermore, pregnancy increases cholesterol levels.[1,2] Thus coronary insufficiency may be aggravated both by hemodynamic changes of pregnancy[3] and elevated cholesterol.[4] Umbilical artery resistance to blood flow is increased in hypercholesterolemia and can lead to fetal growth retardation.[5,6] Recently, increased atherosclerosis progression in offspring of mothers who were hypercholesterolemic during pregnancy was reported.[7]

LDL apheresis has been approved for primary prevention of coronary artery disease in the United States in patients whose LDL-cholesterol remains above 7.77 mmol/l despite maximum tolerated dietary and drug therapy and, for secondary prevention, in patients whose LDL-cholesterol remains above 5.18 mmol/l. There are three reports of LDL apheresis during pregnancy,[8–10] including the present case,[10] and two reports of plasmapheresis to lower LDL during pregnancy.[6,11] In special circumstances – in this case severe coronary artery disease – LDL apheresis therapy may be employed and is safe and efficacious during pregnancy.

References

1. Knopp RH, Warth MR, Carrol CJ. Lipid metabolism in pregnancy. I. Changes in lipoprotein triglyceride and cholesterol in normal pregnancy and the effects of diabetes mellitus. J Reprod Med 1973; 10: 95–101.
2. Desoye G, Schweditsch MO, Pfeiffer KP, Zechner R, Kostner GM. Correlation of hormones with lipid and lipoprotein levels during normal pregnancy and postpartum. J Clin Endocrinol Metab 1987; 64: 704–12.
3. Wallenburg HCS. Maternal haemodynamics in pregnancy. Fet Med Rev 1990; 2: 45–66.
4. Andrews TC, Raby K, Barry J et al. Effect of cholesterol reduction on myocardial ischemia in patients with coronary disease. Circulation 1997; 95: 324–8.
5. Barss V, Phillippe M, Greene MF, Covell L. Pregnancy complicated by homozygous hypercholesterolemia. Obstet Gynecol 1985; 65: 756–7.
6. Beigel Y, Hod M, Fuchs J et al. Pregnancy in a homozygous familial hypercholesterolemic patient treated with long-term plasma exchange. Am J Obstet Gynecol 1990; 162: 77–8.
7. Napoli C, Glass CK, Witztum JL et al. Influence of maternal hypercholesterolaemia during pregnancy on progression of early atherosclerotic lesions in childhood: Fate of Early Lesions in Children (FELIC) study. Lancet 1999; 354: 1234–41.
8. Kroon AA, Swinkels DW, van Dongen PWJ, Stalenhoef AFH. Pregnancy in a patient with homozygous familial hypercholesterolemia treated with long-term low-density lipoprotein apheresis. Metabolism 1994; 43: 1164–70.
9. Teruel JL, Lasuncion MA, Navarro JF, Carrero P, Ortuno J. Pregnancy in a patient with homozygous familial hypercholesterolemia undergoing low-density lipoprotein apheresis by dextran sulfate adsorption. Metabolism 1995; 44: 929–33.
10. Cashin-Hemphill L, Noone M, Abbott JF, Waksmonski CA, Lees RS. Low-density lipoprotein apheresis therapy during pregnancy. Am J Cardiol 2000; 86: 1160.
11. Goldstein BL, Hofschire PJ, Sears TD, Rayburn WF. Long-term plasmapheresis in the homozygous hyperlipidemic patient. Am Heart J 1991; 122: 1465–6.

Case 11
A Case Of Xanthomatous Neuropathy

Gilbert Thompson

History

Miss JC was aged 55 at the time of her referral to Hammersmith Hospital by Professor Neil McIntyre, in 1981. Primary biliary cirrhosis had been diagnosed at the Royal Free Hospital in 1976, when she presented with a brief history of jaundice, pruritus, and weight loss together with widespread cutaneous xanthomas. Her generalized bone pain was attributed to hypertrophic osteoarthropathy and metabolic bone disease, her painful hands and feet to xanthomatous neuropathy.

In 1966 she had been diagnosed with thyrotoxicosis, which was treated medically for 2 years and then by thyroidectomy. Subsequently she remained well until the onset of jaundice in 1975. She was treated with weekly plasma exchanges for 2 months in 1977, without apparent benefit, and then with D-penicillamine but this was discontinued after 6 months because of side effects.

The reason for referral was to attempt to alleviate her hypercholesterolemia and xanthomatous neuropathy by undertaking a course of plasma exchange in conjunction with administration of the experimental HMG-CoA reductase inhibitor, lovastatin (known then as mevinolin). At that stage she was receiving L-thyroxine 0.1 mg and spironolactone 50 mg daily, monthly injections of vitamins A, D, and K, and cholestyramine intermittently.

Physical signs

The patient was thin, with generalized muscle wasting and a BMI of only 17. She was deeply jaundiced and had striking xanthelasma, extensive planar xanthomas of the palms and soles, and gross hepatosplenomegaly. Neurological examination revealed loss of light touch and pain sensation over the fingertips but hyperesthesia to pressure over the proximal phalanges and palms. Tendon reflexes were present and plantar responses were flexor.

Investigations

Hemoglobin was 12 g/dl, with target cells on the blood film. Serum glucose, electrolytes, creatinine, and albumin were all normal but liver function tests were grossly abnormal, with multiple increases above the upper limit of normal in serum bilirubin (>×15), alkaline phosphatase (>×10), aspartate transaminase (>×10), and gamma-glutamyl transpeptidase (>×30).

Fasting serum lipid assay showed a markedly elevated total cholesterol (19.8 mmol/l), slightly raised triglyceride (2 mmol/l), and a markedly reduced HDL-cholesterol (0.34 mmol/l). The presence of Lp-X was demonstrated on agar gel electrophoresis; chromatography of the d1.019–1.063 fraction of ultracentrifuged plasma on Sepharose 4B showed that the ratio of Lp-X:LDL was 4.1. In support of this finding, only 17% of plasma cholesterol was esterified (normal 70%), reflecting the high free cholesterol content of Lp-X.

Management

The patient underwent a course of 21 plasma exchanges at approximately weekly intervals during the first 6 months of 1981, performed with an Aminco continuous flow blood cell separator. The patient was heparinized throughout each procedure, during which 2.4–2.8 l of plasma protein fraction (4.5% human serum albumin) were exchanged vein to vein for an equivalent volume of plasma at a flow rate of 30–40 ml/minute.

Plasma exchange was used alone for 6 weeks, combined with cholestyramine 16 g/day for 3 weeks, and then combined with lovastatin for 10 weeks, the dose gradually being increased from 10 to 50 mg daily. Serum total cholesterol decreased from 18.6 mmol/l before the start of plasma exchange to a mean of 8.4 mmol/l during the period when weekly plasma exchanges were combined with administration of 40–50 mg of lovastatin daily, a reduction of 57%. Mean reductions of 41% and 47%, respectively, were achieved with plasma exchange alone and in combination with cholestyramine.

As shown in Figure 1, lovastatin reduced the post-plasma exchange rate of rebound in cholesterol from 1.5 to 0.9 mmol/l per day, a decrease of 40%. Much of this decrease must have been in Lp-X, as the Lp-X:LDL ratio in plasma fell from 4.1 to 2.6 during lovastatin administration and its cholesterol ester content rose from 17% to 28%. There was no change in triglyceride but HDL-cholesterol rose to 0.63 mmol/l. The patient tolerated plasma exchange and lovastatin well and creatine kinase values remained within the normal range. However, despite an appreciable reduction in the extent of her xanthomas after 6 months treatment there was no improvement in the neuropathic symptoms.

48

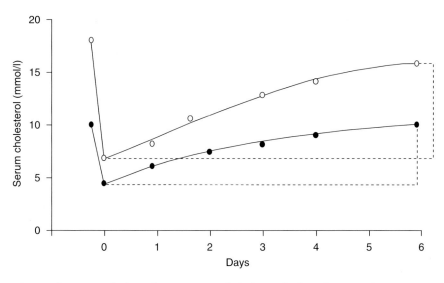

Figure 1 *Rate of rebound in serum total cholesterol after plasma exchange undertaken alone (o) and in conjunction with lovastatin 50 mg/daily (•).*

Discussion

The association of xanthomas and obstructive liver disease was first described by Addison and Gull in 1851, who noted that 'the connection of this affection of the skin with hepatic derangement is obvious'.[1] The severity and distribution of xanthelasma in a postmenopausal woman depicted in their report was strikingly similar to that seen in Miss JC. Patients with marked hypercholesterolemia secondary to chronic biliary obstruction sometimes develop xanthomatous infiltration of the perineurium and endoneurium, resulting in peripheral neuropathy. This can lead to hyperesthesia of sufficient severity as to render it impossible to turn a latch key in the front door, as happened to the subject of this report. Plasma exchange may alleviate this situation, as was shown by Turnberg et al.[2]

The biochemical hallmark of chronic biliary obstruction, Lp-X, results mainly from the spillover of biliary cholesterol and phospholipid into the blood, although diminished lecithin:cholesterol acyltransferase (LCAT) activity may play a contributory role. The largely unesterified cholesterol and phospholipid complex with apolipoprotein C to form discoid particles, which were first termed Lp-X by Seidel et al.[3] The data presented here suggest that HMG-CoA reductase inhibitors reduce Lp-X even more effectively than they do LDL, presumably by reducing the rate of synthesis of its major constituent, free cholesterol, which is often raised in biliary obstruction. However, caution must be exercised when using these drugs in patients with compromised liver function, as they may aggravate the underlying liver disease and increase the risk of iatrogenic myopathy.

Comment

The novel feature of this case report is that it describes the first clinical use of a statin in Britain. The cholesterol-lowering potential of lovastatin had been published only 6 months previously under its original name mevinolin by Alberts et al.[4] and it was their Merck colleague, Dr Jonathan Tobert, who was instrumental in providing supplies of this compound for use on a named patient basis. This arrangement proved to be of major benefit in the treatment of patients with familial hypercholesterolemia at Hammersmith Hospital[5] up until 1989, when simvastatin became the first HMG-CoA reductase inhibitor to be licensed in the UK.

References

1. Addison T, Gull W. On a certain affection of the skin. Vitiligoidea – a, plana b, tuberosa. With remarks and plates. Guys Hospital Reports 1851; 7: 265–76.
2. Turnberg LA, Mahoney MP, Gleeson MH, Freeman CB, Gowenlock AH. Plasmaphoresis and plasma exchange in the treatment of hyperlipaemia and xanthomatous neuropathy in patients with primary biliary cirrhosis. Gut 1972; 13: 976–81.
3. Seidel D, Alaupovic P, Furman RH. A lipoprotein characterizing obstructive jaundice. I. Method for quantitative separation and identification of lipoproteins in jaundiced subjects. J Clin Invest 1969; 48: 1211–23.
4. Alberts AW, Chen J, Kuron G et al. Mevinolin: a highly potent competitive inhibitor of hydroxymethylglutaryl-coenzyme A reductase and a cholesterol-lowering agent. Proc Natl Acad Sci U S A 1980; 77: 3957–61.
5. Thompson GR, Ford J, Jenkinson M, Trayner I. Efficacy of mevinolin as adjuvant therapy for refractory familial hypercholesterolaemia. Q J Med 1986; 60: 803–11.

Case 12
UNUSUALLY SEVERE DOMINANT HYPERCHOLESTEROLEMIA

Rossi Naoumova

The index patient (II,2 on Figure 1A, marked with an arrow), developed angina aged 39 years; his cholesterol was 13.9 mmol/l and premature corneal arcus, very large tendon xanthomata on the dorsum of his hands and Achilles' tendons, and pretibial tuberositas were noted. Two brothers and his father had died of myocardial infarction aged 32 to 62 years. Coronary artery bypass graft (CABG) operation was performed when he was aged 42 and treatment with colestipol was initiated with poor response. In 1985, at the age of 51, he was referred to the Lipid Clinic at Hammersmith Hospital with hypercholesterolemia that was unresponsive to treatment with maximal doses of currently available lipid-lowering drugs (Figure 1B). On a combination of colestipol 30 g/day, bezafibrate 600 mg/day, and nicotinic acid 3 g daily, his fasting total cholesterol was 19.2 mmol/l and triglyceride 3.8 mmol/l, and these levels remained exceptionally high until the introduction of potent statins. During the subsequent 19 years maximal doses of statins in combination with bile acid sequestrants and lately with ezetimibe led to a better control of serum cholesterol and to a decrease in size of his tendon xanthomata; fasting serum triglyceride ranged between 1.5 and 4.72 mmol/l and HDL-cholesterol between 0.7 and 1.1 mmol/l. It is of interest that the patient now follows an exceptionally strict low cholesterol, low-fat diet. He underwent re-do CABG operation in 1994 and has mild peripheral vascular disease and asymptomatic carotid disease. At present the patient remains well with stable angina.

His daughter (III,3) was diagnosed with hypercholesterolemia at the age of 11 years. Her total cholesterol on treatment with colestipol and nicotinic acid was 14.3 mmol/l (pretreatment levels are not known). Currently on treatment with rosuvastatin 40 mg, her total cholesterol is 10.0 mmol/l. The proband's niece (III,1) was referred to the Lipid Clinic at Hammersmith Hospital in 1996 at the age of 38 years with very severe hypercholesterolemia resistant to treatment with statins. She had large Achilles tendon xanthomas and bilateral xanthelasmas on her upper and lower lids, and soft right carotid bruit. On simvastatin 40 mg/day and acipimox 250 mg tds, total cholesterol was 15.5 mmol/l, triglyceride

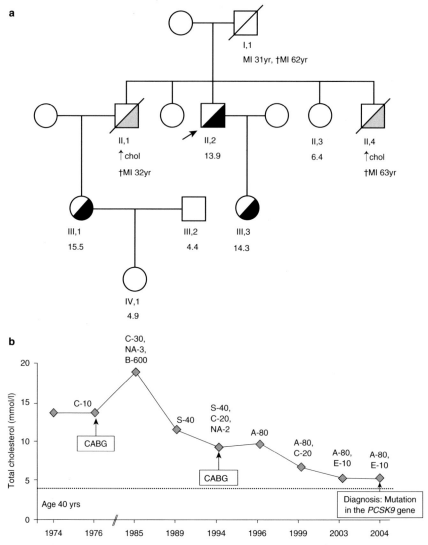

Figure 1 *Family tree (a) and response of the index patient to long-term treatment with lipid-lowering therapy (b). (a). The proband is indicated by an arrow; pretreatment total plasma cholesterol values (mmol/l) are shown below each symbol. Half-shaded symbols indicate known heterozygous carriers of the* PCSK9 *D374Y variant (dark shading) or presumed/obligate carriers (light shading). Some individuals were reported to be hypercholesterolemic, but precise values were not known (↑ chol). † MI, fatal myocardial infarction. (b) The dotted line represents the target total cholesterol concentration that needs to be achieved on treatment. CABG, coronary artery by-pass graft; A, atorvastatin (mg); B, bezafibrate (mg); C, cholestyramine/colestipol (g); E, ezetimibe (mg); NA, nicotinic acid (mg); S, simvastatin (mg).*

1.58 mmol/l, HDL-cholesterol 1.28 mmol/l, and LDL-cholesterol 13.5 mmol/l; on atorvastatin 80 mg her cholesterol remained at 11.3 mmol/l. The patient developed angina in 1997 and coronary angiography showed moderately severe premature coronary artery disease (CAD) and because of her resistance to treatment with statins she underwent partial ileal bypass. In combination with atorvastatin 80 mg and weight loss of 15 kg, this led to a marked decrease in total cholesterol to 5.4 mmol/l, with triglyceride of 1.47 mmol/l and HDL-cholesterol of 0.94 mmol/l. Although the patient subsequently regained 12 kg over the next 4 years, atorvastatin 80 mg maintained her total cholesterol between 6.2 and 7.1 mmol/l, with LDL-cholesterol between 4.2 and 4.8 mmol/l. Recent addition of ezetimibe reduced her total cholesterol to 5.8 mmol/l. She remains well with stable angina.

The affected members of this family have severe autosomal dominant hypercholesterolemia, characterized by elevated levels of total and LDL-cholesterol, tendon xanthomata, and premature atherosclerosis. The best characterized causal genes for this condition, until recently, were the *LDL* receptor and the apolipoproteinB (*apoB*); mutations in these two genes are known to cause familial hypercholesterolemia (FH) and familial defective apoB (FDB), respectively.[1] For nearly 30 years the precise diagnosis in this family was unclear because no mutations in the *LDL receptor* or *apoB* genes were detected. Recently, missense mutations in a third gene, named *PCSK9* (for protein convertase subtilisin/kexin9) have been described to co-segregate with autosomal dominant hypercholesterolemia.[2] We found subsequently that the index patient in the family described here and all his family members who had hypercholesterolemia were heterozygous carriers of the D374Y mutation in the *PCSK9* gene.[3] In addition to this family, we identified two more families of British origin comprising altogether 12 affected individuals. All affected individuals have unusually severe hypercholesterolemia, characterized by very high pretreatment cholesterol levels and early CAD, and they all require somewhat more stringent treatment than typical FH patients, who are heterozygous for defects in the *LDL receptor* or *apoB* genes.[3,4] Despite maximal doses of lipid-lowering drugs and combinations of them (statins plus ezetimibe or bile acid sequestrants), none of our patients with the D374Y missense mutation in the *PCSK9* gene has achieved target cholesterol levels yet. Two of the patients required additional ways to decrease serum cholesterol: chronic LDL apheresis in one patient and partial ileal bypass in patient III,1 (Figure 1A). Perhaps as a result of the severity of the phenotype and maybe because of other yet unknown reasons, the patients seem to be very susceptible to premature CAD. For example, in two of the three families we studied two women died of premature CAD aged 30 and 31 years, respectively.[3]

The *PCSK9* gene encodes a protease named NARC-1 (neutral apoptosis regulated convertase). The role of *PCSK9* has not yet been fully elucidated but there is substantial body of evidence from *in vitro* and *in vivo* studies to suggest that the gene is involved in cholesterol homeostasis by influencing the number of LDL receptors and regulating apoB secretion rate.

In summary, the family presented here has a new form of autosomal dominant hypercholesterolemia, caused by the D374Y missense mutations of the *PCSK9* gene. All the British families we have reported so far,[4] including this one, appear to have an unpredictably severe clinical phenotype, which required early and aggressive lipid-lowering management. The best therapeutic results were achieved when high doses of potent statins were combined with ezetimibe, a cholesterol absorption inhibitor, or bile acid sequestrants. In some cases chronic LDL apheresis or partial ileal bypass were also employed. Early management of the severe hypercholesterolemia is expected to improve prognosis in patients with this disorder, as shown in those with 'classical' FH due to mutations in the *LDL* receptor gene. However, currently available lipid-lowering drugs have improved but not achieved adequate control of serum cholesterol in patients with *PCSK9* mutations. In future, compounds that lead to inhibition of *PCSK9* may have synergistic effect when combined with statins. Nevertheless, despite the lack of precise diagnosis for 30 years the index patient and his affected family members have benefited from the constantly evolving lipid-lowering strategies over the years and have helped us to shed light on a new genetic form of severe hypercholesterolemia.

References

1. Goldstein J, Hobbs H, Brown M. Familial hypercholesterolemia. In: Valle D, Scriver CR, Beaudet A et al., eds. The Metabolic and Molecular Bases of Inherited Disease. New York: McGraw Hill, 2001; 2863–913.
2. Abifadel M, Varret M, Rabes JP et al. Mutations in PCSK9 cause autosomal dominant hypercholesterolemia. Nat Genet 2003; 34: 154–6.
3. Sun XM, Eden ER, Tosi I et al. Evidence for effect of mutant PCSK9 on apolipoprotein B secretion as the cause of unusually severe dominant hypercholesterolaemia. Hum Mol Genet 2005; 14: 1161–9.
4. Naoumova R, Tosi I, Patel D et al. Severe hypercholesterolaemia in four British families with the D374Y mutation in the PCSK9 gene: long-term follow-up and treatment response. Arterioscler Thromb Vasc Biol 2005; 25: 2654–60.

Case 13

A CASE OF EXTREME TRIGLYCERIDEMIA

Richard L Dunbar

A case study

BH is a 42-year-old white gentleman who presented to establish care, reporting a prior history of severe triglyceridemia, with baseline triglycerides over 1000 mg/dl, for which he took simvastatin 80 mg. He has never had pancreatitis and was otherwise healthy and feels fine. His father had peripheral arterial disease, and died from a myocardial infarction (MI) by the age of 68. His mother survived an MI and a cerebrovascular accident (CVA) in her late 60s. His brother survived a CVA at the age of 56. The patient has never smoked, eats a typical Western diet, and alternates between periods of intense exercise to an athletic performance level, and abstinence from physical activity, depending on life circumstances. His blood pressure was 134/78 mm Hg, heart rate 69 beats per minute, weight was 226 pounds, and girth was 44 inches. His physical exam was unremarkable except for the central obesity. Lipids off medication were notable for triglycerides 1105 mg/dl, HDL-cholesterol 26 mg/dl, and total cholesterol of 414 mg/dl (average of four measurements over the previous year). On the statin, the current sample was noted to be lipemic and milky with a creamy layer, with triglycerides 802, HDL-cholesterol 23, and total cholesterol 247. He had high chylomicrons and high VLDL, consistent with type V lipoproteinemia. The triglyceridemia prohibited a reliable approximation of his LDL, but direct measurement of LDL was unnecessary at this stage. Glucose was 100 mg/dl. His Framingham risk score was 8%. He had mild elevations of high-sensitivity C-reactive protein (hsCRP) (2.5 mg/l) and apolipoprotein B (122 mg/dl), and normal LP(a) and homocysteine.

Questions to consider

- What is the goal of therapy for this patient?
- What is his risk of having a cardiovascular event?
- What is the optimal treatment strategy?

Dr Dunbar is supported by an NIH Mentored Patient Oriented Research Award. K12 RRφ17625−φ3.

The American National Cholesterol Education Program (NCEP) provides a detailed and well-reasoned approach to the patient with triglyceride abnormalities in the full version of the Adult Treatment Panel III Report (ATP-III).[1] The NCEP points out that we lack compelling evidence that patients with extremely elevated triglycerides are at higher risk of cardiovascular disease than their peers. It may be the case that the triglycerides of such patients are contained in lipoproteins of such prodigious size that they are incapable of infiltrating the arterial wall, and thus do not increase risk (as reviewed by Dunbar and Rader).[2] On the other hand, when the triglycerides exceed 500 and especially 1000 mg/dl, patients are at risk for pancreatitis from toxic levels of triglycerides. Hence, the foremost concern is acutely lowering triglycerides to avert pancreatitis. Per the NCEP, the goal is to aggressively lower triglycerides to < 500 mg/dl. As it is often impossible to normalize triglycerides, maintenance below 500 mg/dl is seen as a therapeutic success.

Though cardiovascular risk is of lower urgency, this patient does have several other risk factors that suggest that he may indeed have more risk than his peers. There are several guidelines that use scoring systems to arrive at a quantitative prognosis for incident heart disease; for BH, I used the Framingham risk score (FRS).[1] The ATP-III guidelines would count only one major risk factor, low HDL, and his FRS was 8%, suggesting low risk. This means that among a group of nonsmoking men living in Framingham, MA in the 1970s around his age with similar cholesterol and blood pressure, 8% of them had died or had a myocardial infarct by the next decade. A strict reading of the ATP-III report would lead one to consider him low risk. However, the FRS likely underestimates his risk, since it does not consider several softer risk factors, including obesity, ominous family history (albeit, out of the age range), elevated hsCRP, hypertriglyceridemia, and the metabolic syndrome. In practice, it is quite common to see patients whose FRS doesn't seem to match the warning signs from the rest of their history. For this reason the NCEP encourages the physician to modulate the risk upward in the presence of these emerging risk factors.[1,3]

Given that the primary goal is to protect BH from pancreatitis, the physician must appreciate that the statins are among the weakest drugs for lowering triglycerides. Inefficacy of the high-dose statin is not surprising. Three types of nonstatins are preferred by the NCEP, based on their triglyceride-lowering prowess: fibrates, niacin, and fish oil. The bile acid sequestrants are contraindicated because they may raise the triglycerides. The fibrates lower triglycerides between 25 and 50%, niacin 20–40%, and fish oil 30–40%, while statins may lower triglycerides between 7 and 30%.[1]

Initial treatment

Initially, I started BH on high-dose fenofibrate and slowly titrated extended-release niacin. I asked him to take 325 mg of aspirin 30 minutes before taking the niacin. I started the niacin at 500 mg/day and asked him to increase to 1000 mg/day after a month. He returned for follow-up after a month of 1000 mg/day, to check lab work and assess tolerance. At that time lab results indicated triglycerides 422 mg/dl, HDL-cholesterol 39 mg/dl, and total cholesterol 259 mg/dl. He tolerated the medications well, and had started an exercise regimen. I asked him to increase the niacin to 1500 mg/day for another month, and then increase to 2000 mg/day thereafter.

While few patients complain of adverse effects from fibrates, skin flushing from niacin is practically universal. To limit this effect, I asked him to start taking an adult dose of aspirin 30 minutes before taking niacin. I also used the extended-release formulation of niacin, which has a few advantages: (1) the once-daily dose is given at bedtime so that many patients sleep through the flushing effect, (2) the formulation slowly releases niacin, so that flushing is less frequent than with immediate-release niacin, and (3) the medication is regulated by the FDA, which gives considerable assurance of drug quality. The last point is important because supplemental niacin available without prescription often contains no active ingredient.[4] To further limit flushing, I started a low dose of niacin, 500 mg a day, and asked him to titrate slowly by adding 500 mg a month until he reached the target dose of 2000 mg a day.

Follow-up

Over the course of a couple years, I managed BH according to the ATP-III recommendations for severe hypertriglyceridemia, with counseling on diet, exercise, and weight loss. He started an aggressive exercise program, and eventually reached a level of fitness that allowed him to enter a weight-lifting competition. Physical activity enhanced the benefit of combination medication, yielding the following lipid panel: triglycerides 195 mg/dl, HDL-cholesterol 42 mg/dl, LDL-cholesterol 139 mg/dl, and total cholesterol 220 mg/dl. Fasting glucose was 98 mg/dl, rising to 135 mg/dl after a 2-hour glucose tolerance test. He tolerated his medications well, which consisted of fenofibrate 160 mg/day, extended-release niacin 2000 mg/day, and aspirin 325 mg/day.

When the triglycerides are consistently below 500 mg/dl, it is wise to re-evaluate cardiovascular risk and treat as appropriate. When patients reach this point, I consider adding a statin if the patient has moderate to high risk of cardiovascular events (i.e. FRS 10–20% or above 20%, respectively). The optimal cardiovascular prevention strategy for the hypertriglyceridemic population is unknown, though there are data showing that fibrate monotherapy, niacin monotherapy, niacin/fibrate combination therapy, and statin monotherapy reduce coronary heart disease (CHD) events in moderate- to high-risk patients (reviewed by Dunbar and Rader[2]). The patient was not interested in adding a statin, preferring to monitor his status with continued physical exercise. During extended follow-up, the patient's fitness waxed and waned. When he was most sedentary, his triglycerides were in the 400 mg/dl range on the fibrate and niacin, emphasizing the ill effects of torpor. In contrast, the triglycerides normalized when he was at peak performance. Exercise has a remarkable effect on triglyceridemia, and his preference for weight-training suggests a role for strength-building exercise. I selected fenofibrate initially to leave open the possibility of combination with a statin. Because gemfibrozil interferes with the metabolism of statins, that fibrate is more likely to provoke rhabdomyolysis than fenofibrate when paired with a statin. Accordingly the NCEP strongly recommends fenofibrate when contemplating concomitant statin use.[3] For convenience and compliance, if the patient clearly requires a statin in the future, I will keep him on fenofibrate and consider a pill that combines extended-release niacin with lovastatin.

In summary, this patient responded well to combination therapy with a fibrate and niacin, which effectively lowered his triglycerides to a range that protects from pancreatitis. When he added vigorous physical training, he normalized his triglycerides (i.e. < 200 mg/dl) and normalized his HDL (i.e. > 40 mg/dl), so that he no longer met the diagnostic criteria for metabolic syndrome.

References

1. The National Cholesterol Education Program (NCEP) Expert Panel. Third Report of the National Cholesterol Education Program (NCEP) Expert Panel on Detection, Evaluation, and Treatment of High Blood Cholesterol in Adults (Adult Treatment Panel III) Final Report. Circulation 2002; 106(25): 3143–421.
2. Dunbar RL, Rader DJ. Demystifying triglycerides: a practical approach for the clinician. Cleve Clin J Med 2005; 72(8): 661–680.
3. Grundy SM, Cleeman JI, Merz CNB et al. Implications of recent clinical trials for the National Cholesterol Education Program Adult Treatment Panel III Guidelines. Circulation 2004; 110(2): 227–39.
4. Meyers CD, Carr MC, Park S, Brunzell JD. Varying cost and free nicotinic acid content in over-the-counter niacin preparations for dyslipidemia. Ann Intern Med 2003; 139(12): 996–1002.

Case 14

A PATIENT WITH ACUTE SEVERE ABDOMINAL PAIN AND GENERALIZED ERUPTIVE XANTHOMATA

Haralampos J Milionis and Moses S Elisaf

Case history

A 41-year-old man was admitted because of acute, severe central abdominal pain and vomiting. He was a heavy drinker and had smoked about 40 cigarettes/day for the past 20 years. His temperature was 37.2°C, blood pressure 134/82 mm Hg, pulse rate 110 beats/min, and respiration rate 30 breaths/min. He was overweight (BMI of 27 kg/m^2). On examination, generalized *eruptive xanthomata* were observed all over the trunk, back, buttocks, arms, legs (Figure 1a), and knees, while fundoscopy revealed *lipemia retinalis* (Figure 1b). Abdominal distension, tenderness, and absent sounds on auscultation indicated the presence of ileus. An electrocardiogram showed sinus tachycardia, and a chest X-ray was normal. Abdominal films showed a proximal jejunum 'sentinel loop' and a CT scan of the abdomen verified pancreatic inflammation and mild splenomegaly without evidence of gallstones. The appearance of the patient's serum was milky (Figure 1c). Laboratory testing showed leukocytosis (white blood cell count, $11.8 \times 10^3/mm^3$ with 80% neutrophils), serum glucose 480 mg/dl (26.7 mmol/l), creatinine 1.6 mg/dl (141 μmol/l, reference range 53–106 μmol/l), serum sodium 129 mmol/l (reference range 135–145 mmol/l), total cholesterol 830 mg/dl (21.5 mmol/l), triglycerides 8900 mg/dl (100 mmol/l), and HDL-cholesterol 32 mg/dl (0.8 mmol/l). After diluting serum to 'remove' the effect of lipid particles, hyperamylasemia was evident (395 IU/l (upper normal limit, 90 IU/l), while the urine amylase was 5410 IU/l (upper normal limit, 600 IU/l). Arterial pH was 7.2, pCO$_2$ 14 mm Hg, and bicarbonate 6 mmol/l. A urine specimen revealed glycosuria and ketonuria. Agarose gel lipoprotein electrophoresis revealed increased chylomicrons and very-low-density lipoproteins (VLDLs).

With a diagnosis of acute pancreatitis and diabetic ketoacidosis the patient was successfully managed with fluid resuscitation and insulin treatment. On the eighth

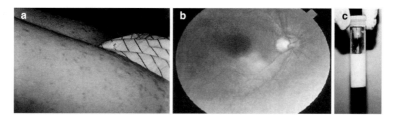

Figure 1 *(a) Generalized eruptive xanthomata on the patient's legs.*
(b) Fundoscopy revealed lipemia retinalis. (c) Milky appearance of the patient's serum.

day of hospitalization he was started on oral fenofibrate 200 mg once daily, and
metformin 850 mg twice daily. Five weeks following admission, the eruptive
xanthomata had regressed and fundoscopy was normal. Upon discharge (day 45),
laboratory evaluation showed: fasting glucose 156 mg/dl (8.7 mmol/l), total
cholesterol 280 mg/dl (7.2 mmol/l), and triglycerides 680 mg/dl (7.7 mmol/l).
The patient was instructed to abstain from alcohol, quit smoking, lose weight, and
follow a strict hypolipidemic diet. At a follow-up visit a year later, the patient was
receiving insulin NPH and oral fenofibrate 200 mg daily. His BMI was 24.5 kg/m^2,
glycosylated hemoglobin 6.9%, and fasting triglycerides 345 mg/dl (3.9 mmol/l),
HDL-cholesterol 29 mg/dl (0.7 mmol/l), and total cholesterol 250 mg/dl
(6.5 mmol/l).

Diagnosis and pathophysiology

This is a case of acute pancreatitis associated with hypertriglyceridemia. The
clinical presentation and laboratory results are most consistent with a type V
hyperlipidemia, Fredrickson class.[1] In contract to type III hyperlipoproteinemia,
the patient lacked skin lesions or tuberosities (e.g. on elbows and knees) and
a beta-band was not evident on agarose gel electrophoresis. Moreover, the
triglyceride to total cholesterol (mg/dl) ratio was 10.7 (usually 8–10:1 for type V
hyperlipoproteinemia, but significantly lower in type III hyperlipoproteinemia).
The patient also had clinical signs consistent with diabetic ketoacidosis and a
history of heavy alcohol intake, both of which can increase triglyceride levels.[2]

The metabolic defect in patients with type V hyperlipoproteinemia can result
from increased and/or decreased catabolism. A diagnosis can be confirmed
by noting the presence of chylomicrons and excess VLDLs on agarose gel
electrophoresis or ultracentrifugal analysis.[1] A simple technique to distinguish
type V from type I hyperlipoproteinemia is to refrigerate the plasma overnight.

Patients with type V hyperlipidemia have a creamy supernatant from chylomicrons and a turbid VLDL-rich infranatant. However, patients with type I hyperlipoproteinemia have a clear infranatant. Most adults with triglycerides >1000 mg/dl (11.3 mmol/l) have type V hyperlipoproteinemia.

Serum triglyceride concentrations >1000 mg/dl (11.3 mmol/l) can be associated with an increased risk of acute pancreatitis.[1,3] Most adults with hyperchylomicronemia have a genetically inherited defect in a factor involved in triglyceride clearance (e.g. heterozygosity for lipoprotein lipase deficiency) coexistent with another condition that is known to raise serum lipids in susceptible individuals. These conditions may include alcohol abuse, obesity, hypothyroidism, pregnancy, estrogen or tamoxifen therapy, glucocorticoid excess, nephrotic syndrome, beta-blocker administration, and diabetes mellitus (diabetes can cause both an overproduction of VLDL and decreased lipoprotein lipase activity).[1,2] The clinical signs and symptoms do not necessarily correlate with the level of hypertriglyceridemia; patients with triglyceride levels as high as 20 000 mg/dl (226 mmol/l) may be asymptomatic, whereas others with a triglyceride level of 3000 mg/dl (33.9 mmol/l) or lower may present with acute pancreatitis.[1,3]

Physical signs. Eruptive xanthomata are characteristic of extreme hypertriglyceridemia. Eruptive xanthomata, consisting of papules with raised yellow centers on the extensor surfaces, especially of the arms and legs, buttocks, and back were prominent in this patient and disappeared within a few weeks on treatment. Eruptive xanthomata are only encountered in patients whose triglycerides exceed at least 2000 mg/dl (22.6 mmol/l), and result from the phagocytosis of chylomicrons by macrophages in the skin. Hepatosplenomegaly is common, and imaging shows 'fatty liver'. Bone marrow biopsy may reveal foam cells. Other features include the white appearance of both the retinal veins and arteries (i.e. lipemia retinalis).

Laboratory evaluation. High triglyceride levels can make the serum appear milky as a result of hyperchylomicronemia. Acute pancreatitis most commonly occurs when serum triglyceride levels exceed 2000–3000 mg/dl (20–30 mmol/l). However, the risk is probably already increased at levels of 500 mg/dl (5.6 mmol/l). The presentation of acute pancreatitis is similar to that arising from other causes. However, increased serum amylase activity may not be detected. Falsely low values may result from assay interference by triglyceride-rich lipoproteins. Removal of chylomicrons from plasma by a brief centrifugation before laboratory tests can eliminate such artefacts.[1]

'Pseudohyponatremia' is another consequence of extreme hypertriglyceridemia, as in the present case. Low serum sodium values are attributed to the inclusion of lipid in the aliquot of blood sampled. When the serum triglycerides exceed 40–50 mmol/l (3500–4500 mg/dl), the concentration of sodium in the aqueous

61

phase (and thus the serum osmolality) may be normal, while spurious serum sodium levels of 120–130 mmol/l are reported. Clinicians should be aware of this condition, since the injudicious infusion of large volumes of isotonic or hypertonic fluids in seriously ill 'hyponatremic' patients with pancreatitis, or uncontrolled diabetes, may be hazardous. This artefact may be obviated with newer methods using ion-selective electrodes for the measurement of electrolytes.

Management

Lifestyle changes. The approach to the patient with type V hyperlipidemia is to modify any predisposing risk factors, as in this patient. Alcohol intake should be limited and diabetes strictly controlled in patients with susceptibility to triglyceride elevation. Obesity is common in all types of hypertriglyceridemia, in which case dietary advice should be directed at weight reduction. In order to lose weight, decreases in overall fat intake may be required. In the case of severe hypertriglyceridemia, when the contribution of chylomicrons is significant, a restriction in all types of fat intake is essential (restriction of daily fat intake to 20 g or below may be necessary). If a patient has elevated triglycerides after lifestyle modification and/or removal of predisposing risk factors, pharmacologic therapy is necessary.[1,2]

Drug therapy. Patients with triglyceride levels > 1000 mg/dl (11.3 mmol/l) should be treated with medication to prevent pancreatitis and the 'chylomicronemia syndrome'.[1] The traditional agents used include fibrates as well as nicotinic acid. The latter is not usually a first-line agent for patients with triglycerides > 1000 mg/dl (11.3 mmol/l), but is usually effective in patients with triglycerides of 500 mg/dl (5.6 mmol/l) or less. Refractory cases may benefit from the addition of a fish oil supplement.

Comment

Treatment is necessary to avoid the risk of acute pancreatitis in extreme hypertriglyceridemia. The association of severe hypertriglyceridemia with ischemic heart disease (IHD) is complex and IHD risk is not necessarily dependent on the triglyceride level. This correlation may be explained by the frequent association of hypertriglyceridemia with obesity, low HDL-cholesterol levels, small dense LDL particles, diabetes mellitus, and peripheral arterial disease in these patients. Therefore, lifestyle modification and appropriate drug treatment may minimize the risk of both acute pancreatitis and vascular disease.

62

References

1. Chait A, Brunzell JD. Chylomicronemia syndrome. Adv Intern Med 1992; 37: 249–73.
2. Chait A, Robertson HT, Brunzell JD. Chylomicronemia syndrome in diabetes mellitus. Diabetes Care 1981; 4: 343–8.
3. Yadav D, Pitchumoni CS. Issues in hyperlipidemic pancreatitis. J Clin Gastroenterol 2003; 36: 54–62.

Case 15

Severe Hypertriglyceridemia Due To Familial Lipoprotein Lipase Deficiency In Pregnancy

John R Burnett and Gerald F Watts

Introduction

Plasma lipid and lipoprotein concentrations are determined by many different environmental and genetic factors. Physiological alterations in maternal lipoprotein metabolism due to estrogen occur during gestation and result in increased plasma concentrations in late term. Maternal hypertriglyceridemia is a characteristic feature during pregnancy, but the exact mechanism remains in doubt.[1] Estrogen concentrations gradually increase during normal pregnancy and during late gestation induce hypertriglyceridemia by increasing the hepatic production and decreasing the peripheral clearance of plasma triglyceride-rich lipoproteins (TRLs).[2] Marked hypertriglyceridemia can develop in the late gestation of pregnancy as a consequence of mutations in genes, such as lipoprotein lipase (LPL) or apolipoprotein E (APOE) or other causes such as diabetes mellitus, alcohol abuse, use of beta-blockers or excessive weight gain.[3,4] Although rarely encountered, severe hypertriglyceridemia may result in the potentially life-threatening complication of acute pancreatitis.[5]

History

The patient was the product of an uneventful term spontaneous vaginal delivery. At age 20 months she presented to her pediatrician with abdominal pain, skin eruptions, and failure to thrive. The patient's blood was noted to be grossly lipemic in appearance and the plasma triglyceride concentration was about 100 mmol/l; predominantly in the chylomicron fraction.

She was placed on a low-fat diet (15% of total calories from fat), which contained medium-chain triglycerides and sufficient corn oil to prevent essential fatty acid deficiency. This regimen resulted in good control of plasma triglyceride

65

levels. Isoelectric focusing with polyacrylamide gel electrophoresis showed that the patient had adequate apoC-II and her *APOE* genotype was e3/3.

At the age of 4 years, post-heparin plasma LPL activity was undetectable, consistent with defective catabolism of TRLs; hepatic lipase activity and very low density lipoprotein (VLDL) apoC-II levels were normal. A diagnosis of chylomicronemia (Fredrickson type I hyperlipoproteinemia) due to familial LPL deficiency was made. Between age 4 and 17 years, while on a low-fat diet (< 20% of dietary energy), the patient's plasma triglyceride concentration fluctuated between 8 and 30 mmol/l. Throughout this period, she maintained normal growth and development. In part, because of satisfactory compliance with a low-fat diet and an active physical lifestyle, she remained asymptomatic and never developed clinical pancreatitis.

At age 21 years, she became pregnant. Because of her previous history, she was kept under strict medical supervision for management of anticipated worsening hypertriglyceridemia during pregnancy and mitigation of high risk of acute pancreatitis.

Examination and investigations

Early in the first trimester her blood pressure was 110/70 mm Hg and there was no proteinuria. There were no eruptive xanthomata and the liver and spleen were not palpable. Fasting plasma glucose, liver and thyroid function tests, and renal biochemistry were all normal. She denied taking alcohol and was lean. Her plasma showed the characteristic appearance of hyperchylomicronemia (Figure 1).

At this time she was screened for an *LPL* gene mutation. The polymerase chain reaction (PCR) method was used to amplify the entire coding region (and exon/intron boundaries) of the subject's *LPL* gene. The patient was found to be a compound heterozygote with both a missense and a nonsense mutation in the *LPL* gene. Studies of her nuclear family confirmed the recessive inheritance of the condition (Figure 2).

Treatment and outcome

Throughout the pregnancy, the patient remained asymptomatic, and had no clinical signs of hyperchylomicronemia, except for occasional lipemia retinalis. A worsening of her plasma triglyceride concentrations occurred in the third trimester, requiring institution of a very-low-fat diet with vitamin A supplementation and intermittent

66

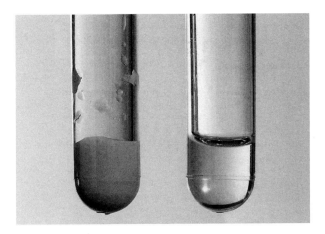

Figure 1 *Plasma from the patient (left) showing the characteristic appearance of hyperchylomicronemia, compared with a normolipidemic control subject (right).*

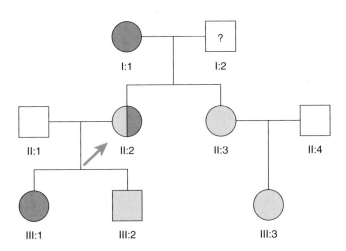

Figure 2 *Pedigree of nuclear kindred showing recessive inheritance. The compound heterozygous patient (II:2) is indicated by the arrow; black, nonsense LPL gene mutation; grey, missense LPL gene mutation; and ?, deceased, not tested (obligate missense LPL gene mutation).*

admissions to hospital for periods of supervised nutritional therapy (Figure 3). She was intolerant of oral intake of medium-chain triglycerides. Both chylomicrons and VLDL contributed to the increased triglyceride levels. Her serum amylase concentrations remained within the reference interval.

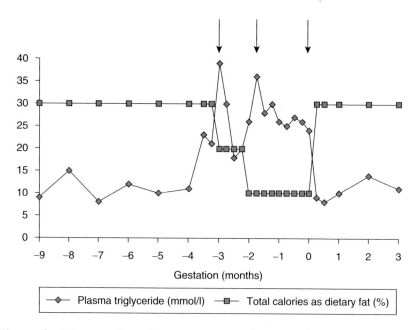

Figure 3   *Plasma triglyceride concentrations and percent of total calories as dietary fat during pregnancy in a patient with familial lipoprotein lipase deficiency. Arrows indicate admissions to hospital.*

At 38 weeks of gestation, the patient went into spontaneous labor and she delivered a healthy 3.3 kg female infant. A fasting plasma triglyceride concentration immediately post-partum fell to < 10 mmol/l.

Commentary

Plasma triglyceride concentrations normally rise during the third trimester of pregnancy by two- to three-fold due to both an estrogen-induced increase in hepatic VLDL secretion and a decrease in LPL activity.[1,2] This physiological increase in plasma triglyceride concentration, with a peak at 2.26–3.39 mmol/l, is thought to have little consequence.[6] However, more marked increases in triglyceride have been reported in association with partial and markedly reduced or absent LPL activity and with the apoE2 isoform with variable pregnancy outcomes.[7–12] Severe hypertriglyceridemia during pregnancy when complicated by acute pancreatitis carries a significant risk of morbidity and mortality for the mother and mortality for the fetus.[5]

LPL (EC 3.1.1.34) is the rate-determining enzyme in the hydrolysis of the triglyceride core in circulating TRLs. LPL belongs to a family that includes hepatic lipase, pancreatic lipase, and the recently discovered endothelial lipase. Catalytically active LPL is a noncovalent homodimeric glycoprotein anchored to heparin sulfate proteoglycans on the luminal plasma membrane of capillary endothelium, where it acts on TRLs delivering free fatty acids to parenchymal cells.[13]

Familial LPL deficiency (OMIM 238600) is a rare recessive disorder characterized by severe hypertriglyceridemia due to the accumulation in plasma of TRLs that result from an absence of LPL activity. The population frequency is one per million people with a carrier frequency of about one in 500.[13-15] Patients with familial LPL deficiency often have extremely low or absent LPL activity in post-heparin plasma. This disorder is usually detected in childhood based on repeated episodes of abdominal pain, pancreatitis, eruptive xanthomata, and hepatosplenomegaly. The severity of the symptoms is proportional to the degree of chylomicronemia, which in turn is dependent on dietary fat intake. Obligate heterozygotes are usually asymptomatic, but can have up to a 50% decrease in post-heparin LPL activity and variable plasma triglyceride concentrations.

The human *LPL* gene located on chromosome 8p22, spans more than 35 kb, contains 10 exons, and codes for a mature protein of 448 amino acids. Numerous structural mutations in the *LPL* gene have been reported to be associated with a catalytically defective LPL protein.[14] Familial LPL-deficient individuals are either homozygous for a single mutation or are compound heterozygotes. Most mutations that cause LPL deficiency, as in this patient, are either missense or nonsense and are clustered in the region coded by exons 4, 5, and 6, which forms the proposed catalytic domain of LPL. Another genetic cause of chylomicronemia is due to deficiency or absence of apoC-II, a co-factor necessary for normal activation of LPL. This later genetic etiology was excluded in our patient, but would not appreciably have altered our medical management of her metabolic disorder.

The management of severe hypertriglyceridemia in pregnancy with familial LPL deficiency involves prevention of pancreatitis in the mother and delivery of a healthy baby. Successful pregnancy outcome has been reported in patients with familial LPL deficiency using dietary fat restriction with the aim to keep the plasma triglyceride concentration < 10–15 mmol/l; use of parenteral nutrition,[10] extracorporeal removal of plasma lipids, fibrates, and n-3 fatty acids have also been described.[11,16,17] Ideally, pre-conception counselling should occur with the aim to optimize plasma triglyceride concentrations by adherence to a low-fat diet. This should involve referral or co-management with a physician with a special interest in lipid disorders. It is also paramount that a specialist dietician is involved to ensure that correct nutrient balance and composition is achieved; use of medium-chain triglycerides that are not metabolized via LPL and vitamin A supplementation are important. Nutritional supplementation with n-3 fatty acids may also be used safely,[16] but was not employed in this patient who found taking

69

the high doses required very unpalatable. Frequent monitoring of plasma triglyceride levels throughout pregnancy will allow early detection of significant hypertriglyceridemia and, as in our patient, initiation of treatment strategies to avoid complications.

It is estimated that pregnancy-associated hypertriglyceridemia is the cause of 4–6% of all episodes of pancreatitis during pregnancy. In our opinion, a patient with familial LPL deficiency should be admitted to hospital if abdominal pain occurs or if plasma triglyceride concentration exceeds 40 mmol/l. In this setting, the patient should, as in our case, be placed on a very-low-fat diet and if required intravenous glucose support until resolution of symptoms. Subsequently, a very-low-fat diet (< 15% of calories) should be instituted, being careful to avoid essential fatty acid deficiency. With acute pancreatitis, a conservative approach involving standard analgesia, parenteral glucose therapy, and intravenous heparin may initially be attempted, but very severe cases will respond well to extracorporeal lipid removal employing, for example, plasmapheresis.[17] We do not consider there is a safe place for prolonged use of heparin and fibrates or nicotinic acid in pregnancy-associated hypertriglyceridemia.[18] The use of high-dose antioxidants and an insulin infusion to treat severe hypertriglyceridemia and prevent pancreatitis in nondiabetics has also been described, but there is no published experience in pregnancy.[19,20]

Women with LPL deficiency should preferably not breast-feed since absence of the enzyme in mammary tissue results in nutritionally deficient milk. Estrogen-containing contraceptives and clomiphene should also be avoided since they exacerbate hypertriglyceridemia and increase the risk of pancreatitis.[21]

What have I learnt from this case?

Maternal hypertriglyceridemia is a characteristic feature during pregnancy. Severe hypertriglyceridemia can develop in the late gestation of pregnancy as a consequence of mutations in genes such as *LPL* and in some cases, extremely high triglyceride concentrations may result in acute pancreatitis. Severe hypertriglyceridemia during pregnancy, especially when complicated with pancreatitis, carries a significant risk of mortality for both the mother and the fetus. Management of severe hypertriglyceridemia in pregnancy with familial LPL deficiency involves prevention of pancreatitis in the mother and delivery of a healthy baby. Early referral to a lipid specialist and a dietitian, and education of the patient and family will avoid this complication and the need for radical therapy, such as plasmapheresis.

References

1. Knopp RH, Bergilin RO, Wahl PW et al. Population-based lipoprotein lipid reference values for pregnant women compared to nonpregnant women classified by sex hormone usage. Am J Obstet Gynecol 1982; 143: 626–37.

2. Alvarez JJ, Montelongo A, Iglesias A, Lasunción MA, Herrera E. Longitudinal study on lipoprotein profile, high density lipoprotein subclass, and postheparin lipases during gestation in women. J Lipid Res 1996; 37: 299–308.

3. Ma Y, Liu MS, Ginzinger D et al. Gene-environment interaction in the conversion of a mild-to-severe phenotype in a patient homozygous for a $Ser^{172} \rightarrow Cys$ mutation in the lipoprotein lipase gene. J Clin Invest 1993; 91: 1953–8.

4. McGladdery SH, Frohlich JJ. Lipoprotein lipase and apoE polymorphisms: relationship to hypertriglyceridemia during pregnancy. J Lipid Res 2001; 42: 1905–12.

5. De Chalain TMB, Michell WL, Berger GMB. Hyperlipidemia, pregnancy and pancreatitis. Surg Gynecol Obstet 1988; 167: 469–73.

6. Salameh WA, Mastrogiannis DS. Maternal hyperlipidemia in pregnancy. Clin Obstet Gynecol 1994; 37: 66–77.

7. Watts GF, Cameron J, Henderson A, Richmond W. Lipoprotein lipase deficiency due to long-term heparinization presenting as severe hypertriglyceridemia in pregnancy. Postgrad Med J 1991; 67: 1062–4.

8. Watts GF, Morton K, Jackson P, Lewis B. Management of patients with severe hypertriglyceridemia during pregnancy: report of two cases with familial lipoprotein lipase deficiency. Br J Obstet Gynaecol 1992; 99: 163–6.

9. Hsia SH, Connelly PW, Hegele RA. Successful outcome in severe pregnancy-associated hyperlipidemia: a case report and literature review. Am J Med Sci 1995; 309: 213–18.

10. Henderson H, Leisegang F, Hassan F, Hayden M, Marais D. A novel Glu421Lys substitution in the lipoprotein lipase gene in pregnancy-induced hypertriglyceridemic pancreatitis. Clin Chim Acta 1998; 269: 1–12.

11. Al-Shali K, Wang J, Fellows F et al. Successful pregnancy outcome in a patient with severe chylomicronemia due to compound heterozygosity for mutant lipoprotein lipase. Clin Biochem 2002; 35: 125–30.

12. Ma Y, Ooi TC, Liu MS et al. High frequency of mutations in the human lipoprotein lipase gene in pregnancy-induced chylomicronemia: possible association with apolipoprotein E2 isoform. J Lipid Res 1994; 35: 1066–75.

13. Merkel M, Eckel RH, Goldberg IJ. Lipoprotein lipase: genetics, lipid uptake, and regulation. J Lipid Res 2002; 43: 1997–2006.

14. Hayden MR, Ma Y. Molecular genetics of human lipoprotein lipase deficiency. Mol Cell Biochem 1992; 113: 171–6.

15. Santamarina-Fojo S. The familial chylomicronemia syndrome. Endocrinol Metab Clin North Am 1998; 27: 551–67.

16. Glueck CJ, Streicher P, Wang P, Sprecher D, Fako JM. Treatment of severe familial hypertriglyceridemia during pregnancy with very-low-fat diet and n-3 fatty acids. Nutrition 1996; 12: 202–5.

17. Lennertz A, Parhofer KG, Samtleben W, Bosch T. Therapeutic plasma exchange in patients with chylomicronemia syndrome complicated by acute pancreatitis. Ther Apher 1999; 3: 227–33.

18. Yen TH, Chang CT, Wu MS, Huang CC. Acute rhabdomyolysis after gemfibrozil therapy in a pregnant patient complicated with acute pancreatitis and hypertriglyceridemia while receiving continuous veno-venous hemofiltration therapy. Ren Fail 2003; 25: 139–43.

19. Heaney AP, Sharer N, Rameh B, Braganza JM, Durrington PN. Prevention of recurrent pancreatitis in familial lipoprotein lipase deficiency with high-dose antioxidant therapy. J Clin Endocrinol Metab 1999; 84: 1203–5.

20. Jabbar MA, Zuhri-Yafi MI, Larrea J. Insulin therapy for a non-diabetic patient with severe hypertriglyceridemia. J Am Coll Nutr 1998; 17: 458–61.

21. Castro MR, Nguyen TT, O'Brien T. Clomiphene-induced severe hypertriglyceridemia and pancreatitis. Mayo Clin Proc 1999; 74: 1125–8.

Case 16

MANAGING COMBINED HYPERLIPOPROTEINEMIA IN A MAN WITH THE METABOLIC SYNDROME

Paul Nestel

Clinical history

Visit 1. A 54-year-old man presented because his brother had a heart attack aged 52 years. An aunt had diabetes. He had been overweight since his 40s although at 85 kg did not consider weight a problem. He had had an attack of gout 6 years ago. His blood pressure had been 'under observation'. He was a nonsmoker, played golf at weekends, and worked long hours in a sedentary occupation.

He 'ate well' within a fairly routine pattern of eating, comprising eggs and buttered toast for breakfast, ham and cheese sandwiches for lunch, and 'meat and veg' at night. He was not a sweet eater but enjoyed cheese, rarely ate fish and avoided vegetarian dishes. Alcohol consumption averaged two beers after work and a glass or two of wine with dinner.

He was surprised at his waist circumference, 103 cm ('my trousers fit'), and that his BMI was $30.2 \, \text{kg/m}^2$. Clinical examination showed no cardiovascular abnormality (heart, carotids, peripheral pulses) other than elevated blood pressure, 152/96. The liver was not palpable and no xanthomata were evident. A resting electrocardiogram was normal.

Clinical chemistry revealed dyslipidemia, insulin resistance, hepatic steatosis, and hyperuricemia. Fasting plasma lipids (mmol/l): total cholesterol, 6.70; triglyceride, 3.62; HDL-cholesterol, 0.82; calculated LDL-cholesterol, 4.21. Blood glucose (fasting): 6.8 mmol/l; 2 hours after 75 g glucose drink: 8.9 mmol/l. Plasma urate: 0.50 mmol/l. Liver function tests showed abnormal gamma glutamyl transferase (γGT): 368 (normal < 60 U/l), reflecting hepatic steatosis or excess hepatic triglyceride, commonly seen in the metabolic syndrome and also with alcohol excess.

Hypertension, impaired glucose tolerance (insulin resistance), and combined dyslipidemia, together with overweight and abdominal adiposity fit the diagnostic criteria of the metabolic syndrome. Hyperuricemia is not uncommon with the syndrome.

Initial considerations. His absolute risk for future clinical coronary heart disease (CHD) based on the algorithm derived from the Framingham database was > 20% over the next 10 years. In addition, the presence of four components of the metabolic syndrome heightens that risk, as shown in the West of Scotland Coronary Prevention Study (WOSCOPS)[1] in which the risks for both future cardiovascular events and type 2 diabetes increased with the number of metabolic syndrome components. A 'risk chart' was discussed with the patient. At this stage, no further investigations seemed warranted.

Initial clinical management

The initial management in an asymptomatic individual should focus on changing the energy balance by reducing food intake and increasing physical activity. He was relieved to learn that modest weight loss based on an eating pattern with 'which he could live' plus regular moderate physical exertion such as taking a brisk half-hour walk on most days during his lunch break, might suffice initially. The trials[2] that supported this advice were discussed.

Further considerations. The optimal mixture of macronutrients that best achieves weight loss and improvement in cardiovascular risk is debatable. The patient requested but was discouraged from an Atkins-type diet and was shown the result of a recent trial that compared several weight loss diets, all of which were found to lead to similar weight losses after 1 year.[3] The key principle of the traditional weight loss diet emphasizes reducing fat intake from foods that are rich in saturated fat and cholesterol. Foods that contain slowly digested carbohydrates and hence slowly absorbed glucose are preferable to rapidly digestible starches. There appears to be an additional benefit in restricting carbohydrates in subjects with the metabolic syndrome in that insulin sensitivity is thus more readily restored. If both carbohydrates and fats are to be reduced proportionately more than their contribution to energy restriction then protein must be proportionately increased. Raising the protein content of a weight loss diet improves insulin sensitivity and limits the loss of muscle. Eating very lean, small cuts of meat, low-fat dairy products, whole-grain cereals, fruits, vegetables, and fish was therefore the basis of advice given to the patient. Alcohol intake was limited to one drink daily. Salt consumption was restricted. A guide was provided that identified foods of choice and foods to be avoided or restricted. Advice from a dietitian was not regarded as essential at this point.

Response to initial management

Visit 2. The patient was seen after 8 weeks when he had lost 6.5 kg weight and 1.5 cm around the waist. He found the lifestyle recommendations compatible.

Clinical chemistry showed some improvement. Concentrations of fasting plasma lipids (mmol/l): total cholesterol, 6.16; triglyceride, 2.95; LDL-cholesterol, 4.08. Blood glucose (6.4 mmol/l) had improved, as had the blood pressure (148/92). Lower γGT (275 U/l) indicated less hepatic fat. However, the urate level rose to 0.54 mmol/l and HDL-cholesterol fell to 0.73 mmol/l. HbA1c, an index of long-term glucose homeostasis, was normal at 5.8%. The rationale for this test as well as for microalbuminuria (also normal) was to provide a baseline should the impaired glucose tolerance progress to diabetes.

Further considerations. The improvements were in line with expectation. Although some individuals fare better others show disappointing results after modest weight loss. The rise in urate with weight loss occasionally precipitates gout. An initial reduction in HDL-cholesterol following acute weight loss is not unusual. The HDL concentration may remain disappointingly low even when other lipids return to normal levels.

This was one of several considerations that led to pharmacological intervention at this stage (see Table 1). It seemed unlikely that his lipid profile would improve sufficiently to reduce the risk for cardiovascular events. The issue then became whether a statin or a fibrate should be the initial drug of choice. Subgroup analyses of patients with the metabolic syndrome in both the Heart Protection Study (HPS) and the Scandinavian Simvastatin Survival Study (4S)[4] revealed a favorable reduction in cardiovascular events. On the other hand a similar group of patients with insulin resistance in the Veterans Administration Trial (VA HIT) also benefited favorably from treatment with gemfibrozil. Since this patient's LDL concentration remained high he was initially treated with simvastatin 40 mg (after a run-in with 20 mg) daily. The possibility of myalgia and arthralgia was stressed and a baseline assessment was quickly made of such current ailments.

Visit 3. Two months later the patient had lost a further 3 kg weight and 1 cm around the waistline. His blood pressure was virtually normal (138/86) and plasma lipids (mmol/l) were found to have improved further with the exception of the HDL-cholesterol concentration. Total cholesterol, 5.0; triglyceride, 2.42; HDL-cholesterol, 0.77; LDL-cholesterol, 3.12. Glucose was borderline (6.0 mmol/l).

In view of the persistently low HDL-cholesterol as well as of hypertriglyceridemia and continuing, albeit lower risk, fenofibrate was added to the treatment. Although the risk of myopathy is only marginally, if at all, increased with a fenofibrate/simvastatin combination, the dose of simvastatin was reduced to 20 mg daily.

75

Table 1   Steps taken in managing dyslipidemia in the metabolic syndrome

Problem	Issues	Treatment options
Visceral obesity	Waist circumference is best index	Weight loss by reducing fat and carbohydrate and a
	Lifestyle changes initially	relative increase in protein
	Physical activity	Moderate aerobic 5 × weekly
Combined dyslipidemia	Assess absolute risk	If high consider drug therapy
	High LDL predominates	Begin with a statin
	High triglyceride plus low HDL predominates	Consider fibrate first
	Lipid targets not met	Combine statin and fibrate
	If LDL still above target	Add ezetimibe
	If triglyceride/HDL remains a major concern	Substitute niacin for fibrate
	In all combination therapy be alert to note adverse effects	
Insulin resistance	Therapy that assists managing dyslipidemia	Consider metformin
Hypertension	Avoid drugs that worsen dyslipidemia or insulin sensitivity	Consider ACE inhibitors

Visit 4. His weight had now stabilized at 76 kg but waist circumference was still 99 cm, indicating that he should persist with the dietary regime, although he could now eat a little more and indulge in an occasional doubling of alcohol intake. Blood pressure rose as weight stabilized and at 150/94 required specific treatment; 4 mg daily perindopril was prescribed. In view of the insulin-resistant state and persistent low HDL-cholesterol an ACE inhibitor was preferred to a low-dose diuretic.

The lipid profile improved further and approached target values suggested in current guidelines. Fasting plasma lipids (mmol/l): total cholesterol, 4.58; triglyceride, 1.66; HDL-cholesterol, 0.94; LDL-cholesterol, 2.88. Glucose was normal at 5.9 mmol/l and γGT declined to 168 U/l.

Further considerations. The additional options to lower LDL-cholesterol to < 2.6 mmol/l included raising simvastatin to 40 mg and/or adding ezetimibe (an inhibitor of cholesterol absorption), especially as a single combination tablet of simvastatin with ezetemibe would soon become available. In the interim, the dose of simvastatin was increased to 40 mg daily, since the patient had experienced no adverse effects and liver function tests (other than γGT) and creatine kinase (CK) were normal after combined therapy.

Visit 5. Without further weight change, blood pressure became normal with perindopril therapy (132/78) and LDL-cholesterol fell to target level. Total cholesterol, 4.1 mmol/l; triglyceride, 1.52 mmol/l; HDL-cholesterol, 0.98 mmol/l; LDL-cholesterol, 2.42 mmol/l. Urate concentration had fallen to 0.48 mmol/l and no specific prophylactic treatment was considered since he had suffered only one attack of gout and renal function was normal.

Further plans were to encourage the lifestyle changes that had led to initial improvement and to advise his general practitioner to monitor blood pressure and lipids at regular intervals. The patient was discharged from the clinic with his absolute risk halved.

References

1. Sattar N, Gaw A, Scherbakova O et al, Metabolic syndrome with and without C-reactive protein as a predictor of coronary heart disease and diabetes in the West of Scotland Coronary Prevention Study. Circulation 2003; 108: 414–19.

2. Diabetes Prevention Program Research Group. Reduction in the incidence of type 2 diabetes with lifestyle intervention and metformin. N Engl J Med 2002; 346: 393–403.

3. Dansinger MJ, Gleason JA, Griffith JL, Selker HP, Schaefer EJ. Comparison of the Atkins, Ornish, Weight Watchers, and Zone diets for weight loss and heart disease risk reduction: a randomized trial. JAMA 2005; 293: 43–53.

4. Ballantyne CM, Olsson AG, Cook TJ et al. Influence of high-density lipoprotein cholesterol and elevated triglyceride on coronary heart disease events and response to simvastatin therapy in 4S. Circulation 2001; 104: 3046–51.

Case 17

LIPID THERAPY FOR DYSLIPIDEMIA IN THE PRESENCE OF THE METABOLIC SYNDROME

Sander J Robins

Patient profile

Sam is a 67-year-old man with a history of an uncomplicated myocardial infarction (MI) at age 55 years and an ischemic stroke 3 months ago that has left him with slight left upper arm weakness. Aside from the stroke Sam believes his recent general health has been good. However, since his MI he has become increasingly sedentary and gained appreciable weight. He describes multiple attempts to lose weight, employing different kinds of diets, without much success. For the past 3 years Sam has been treated with a statin because a doctor, a specialist, told him that his cholesterol was too high.

The patient currently experiences some shortness of breath but denies angina or leg pains upon walking. He has never smoked and says that his cholesterol values have always been low and now with statin therapy are even lower. He says he did have a mild increase in his blood pressure before his stroke but that with blood pressure medicine his blood pressure is now okay. He has no history of diabetes, and no family history of diabetes, heart disease, or stroke. In addition to therapy with the statin, atorvastatin 20 mg/day, and a thiazide diuretic, the patient now also regularly takes an antiplatelet drug.

Sam's exam was notable for obesity with a BMI of $31.5 \, kg/m^2$ and a waist circumference of 108 cm. His blood pressure was 130/85. His cardiovascular exam was normal and his neurologic exam revealed only left upper extremity weakness.

His blood chemistries were obtained after he had fasted for about 10 hours and showed the following: total cholesterol, 157 mg/dl (desirable range < 200 mg/dl); LDL-cholesterol, 90 mg/dl (< 100 mg/dl); HDL-cholesterol 31 mg/dl (> 40 mg/dl (men)); triglycerides, 180 mg/dl (< 150 mg/dl); Total cholesterol/HDL-cholesterol, 5.07 (< 5.00); glucose 118 mg/dl (< 100 mg/dl).

79

Underlying pathology: the metabolic syndrome and insulin resistance

With high triglycerides and a low HDL-cholesterol this patient has what traditionally has been labeled a 'dyslipidemia'. However, with an increase also in waist circumference, blood pressure, and glucose in conjunction with abormalities in triglycerides and HDL-cholesterol this patient has all five of the criteria that characterize the metabolic syndrome, as defined by NCEP, ATP-III.[2] The metabolic syndrome appears to be increasing in frequency (especially in the Western world) in parallel with increasing obesity and is clearly associated with an increased risk of major cardiac events and stroke. Notably, a high cholesterol or, more specifically a high LDL-cholesterol, is not a component of the metabolic syndrome and, indeed, levels of LDL-cholesterol with the metabolic syndrome are often in a relatively low range.

Although there is much discussion as to what constitutes the underlying pathology of the metabolic syndrome, a prime candidate is insulin resistance. Insulin resistance almost always occurs in the presence of obesity (with, especially, an increase in visceral fat) and underlies the development of type 2 diabetes, long known to be associated with a dyslipidemia and an increase in cardiovascular (CV) events. Moreover, not only is diabetes with underlying insulin resistance associated with an increase in CV events but even without type 2 diabetes, insulin resistance has been independently associated with an increased incidence of CV events.

Therapy for dyslipidemia in the presence of the metabolic syndrome and insulin resistance

Who is insulin resistant? In clinical practice we can most often make a judgment that a patient like Sam is likely to be insulin resistant. Although insulin measurements are not standardized and probably should not be used in clinical practice to diagnose insulin resistance, Reaven[1] has advocated using the triglyceride/ HDL-cholesterol ratio which, when ≥ 3.5, appears to be as sensitive as high plasma insulin levels in identifying the patient with insulin resistance Sam's triglyceride/HDL-cholesterol ratio was 5.8.

Options for therapy for dyslipidemia (... especially with insulin resistance). There is overwhelming consensus that cholesterol (i.e. LDL-cholesterol) should be the

80

prime target of lipid therapy. However, in the case of the patient with a rather profound dyslipidemia who has a low cholesterol (albeit, in the case of Sam presumably due in some part to statin therapy), a strong case might be made for the priority of lipid therapy that is known to primarily normalize triglycerides and HDL-cholesterol. Here, the traditional choices have been therapy with a fibrate or niacin. Here also, we have much less secure evidence from clinical trials than with statin therapy for high cholesterol that a fibrate, niacin, or even a statin would be most likely to reduce CV events.

A central question in this discussion is the following: what is the evidence that like cholesterol lowering with statins, the *clinical benefit* of any lipid drug for a dyslipidemia (especially in the presence of insulin resistance) is dependent on (or primarily correlated with) the *magnitude* of triglyceride lowering and/or HDL-cholesterol raising? The short answer to this question is simply this: at present there is no evidence that clinical CV event reduction with therapy to correct a dyslipidemia is analogous to therapy to lower a high cholesterol, i.e. is dependent on the magnitude of change in lipids or achieving certain 'normal' values of lipids. Indeed, in VA-HIT (Veterans Affairs HDL Intervention Trial)[3] therapy with the fibrate, gemfibrozil, was shown to significantly reduce major CV events (MI, CHD death, and stroke) in individuals with a dyslipidemia and a low LDL-cholesterol, although this therapy produced: (1) no reduction in LDL-cholesterol, (2) a relatively small increase in HDL-cholesterol (from a mean of 32 to 34 mg/dl), and (3) a decrease in triglycerides that, however, failed to predict a significant reduction in CV events.

VA-HIT also demonstrated[4] that at equivalent levels of low HDL-cholesterol (see Figure 1) or levels of high triglycerides (data not shown): (1) major coronary events were more frequent with insulin resistance than without insulin resistance regardless of the level of HDL-cholesterol and (2) that a reduction in coronary events with fibrate therapy was more profound in the presence of insulin resistance than without insulin resistance.

We have no information at present from any of the large clinical endpoint trials that statin therapy will effectively reduce CV events in individuals with relatively low levels of cholesterol coupled with insulin resistance. Furthermore, although niacin is generally regarded as a more potent HDL-cholesterol raising drug than either a fibrate or a statin, niacin is well known to increase blood glucose levels and may increase insulin resistance.

What to do? Unfortunately, no trials have been conducted to directly compare the clinical efficacy of various classes of lipid drugs in the patient like Sam with a low cholesterol and a dyslipidemia – especially with a dyslipidemia that is associated with obesity and probable insulin resistance.

Drugs like statins and fibrates have multiple lipid and nonlipid (i.e. pleiotropic) effects. In a case like Sam's one might feel justified in not changing therapy and, in

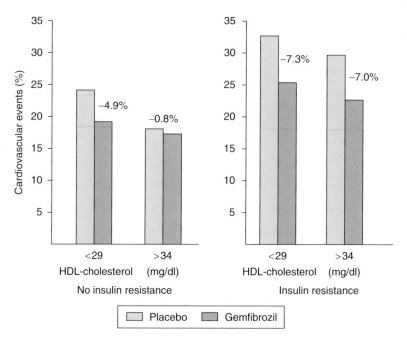

Figure 1   *Effect of gemfibrozil on cardiovascular events in the presence or absence of insulin resistance. Data from VA-HIT,[4] a 5-year placebo-controlled clinical endpoint trial with the fibrate, gemfibrozil, showing (1) the effect of insulin resistance (as assessed by the HOMA calculation) on the development of MI, stroke, or cardiac death at different levels of HDL-C (HDL-cholesterol) and (2) the effect of gemfibrozil therapy on these endpoints with and without insulin resistance at different levels of HDL-C. Groups taking placebo or gemfibrozil are separated into the lowest and highest tertile levels of HDL of <29 mg/dl and >34 mg/dl in VA-HIT. The absolute difference in events with gemfibrozil compared with placebo is shown by the percentage values associated with each set of bars.*

spite of his recent stroke, it might be asked 'should one continue to treat Sam with a statin?'. Alternatively, citing the results of VA-HIT, one might make a strong case for adding a fibrate to Sam's therapy or even discontinuing statin therapy in favor of a fibrate. Finally, another possibility would be to use insulin-sensitizing therapy with a thiazolidinedione (TZD) with or without traditional lipid drug therapy to reduce CV risk. Although these drugs are known to modestly increase HDL-cholesterol and decrease triglyceride levels, there are no clinical trials at present to indicate that this class of drugs will decrease CV events.

A perspective

The patient like Sam is apt to be more prevalent in the future with a worldwide increase in obesity. Lipid therapy for dyslipidemia may not be as straightforward as reducing high cholesterol and therapeutic decisions need be based, when possible, on clinical trial data not a paradigm that is mostly related to the CV benefit that derives from cholesterol-lowering therapy.

References

1. Expert Panel on Detection, Evaluation, and Treatment of High Blood Cholesterol in Adults. Executive Summary of the Third Report of the National Cholesterol Education Program (NCEP) Expert Panel on Detection, Evaluation, and Treatment of High Blood Cholesterol in Adults (Adult Treatment Panel III). JAMA 2001; 285: 2486–97.
2. Reaven G. Metabolic syndrome. Pathophysiology and implications for management of cardiovascular disease. Circulation 2002; 106: 286–8.
3. Robins SJ, Collins D, Wittes JT et al. Relation of gemfibrozil treatment and lipid levels with major coronary events: VA-HIT: a randomized controlled trial. JAMA 2001; 285: 1585–91.
4. Robins SJ, Rubins HB, Faas FH et al. on behalf of the VA-HIT Study Group. Insulin resistance and cardiovascular events with low high-density lipoprotein cholesterol: the Veterans Affairs HDL Intervention Trial (VA-HIT). Diabetes Care 2003; 26: 1513–17.

Case 18

FAMILIAL COMBINED HYPERLIPIDEMIA: THE CASE OF TRIGLYCERIDES

Manuel Castro Cabezas and Ton J Rabelink

The case

Mr B is a 40-year-old man who was referred to our Lipid Clinic for diagnosis and treatment of combined hyperlipidemia. He had never been ill before and laboratory measurements had been done only at medical screenings for his mortgage. He did not know his cholesterol levels. He did not smoke and did not drink any alcohol at all. He was director of his own company and had no time for sport. He was married and the couple were thinking of extending the family, but there were no children yet. He had visited his general practitioner to have his cholesterol checked. His brother, who was 2 years older, had recently suffered a myocardial infarction and a high cholesterol level had been found by his cardiologist. He had been advised to have his relatives screened for high cholesterol and for this purpose Mr B visited his general practitioner (GP). At laboratory screening by the GP, his cholesterol was 6.8 mmol/l, fasting triglycerides 9.5 mmol/l, and HDL-cholesterol 0.78 mmol/l. This lipid profile and the family history motivated the GP to refer Mr B to our Lipid Clinic.

Exploring the family history of Mr B, it appeared that his father had died suddenly at the age of 58 and that his father's father had suffered a stroke at the age of 60. One brother and one sister of Mr B's father had also had cardiac problems and were using lipid-lowering drugs.

Physical examination showed a healthy male without signs of hyperlipidemia (no xanthomas, and thin Achilles tendons; no arcus lipoides or xanthelasmata). His blood pressure was 170/85. He was 1.80 m tall and his body weight was 91 kg. His waist circumference was 105 cm. Laboratory tests revealed a combined hyperlipidemia with total cholesterol of 6.45 mmol/l and fasting triglycerides of 5.61 mmol/l. His HDL-cholesterol was 0.91 and his apolipoprotein B (apoB) was 1.26 g/l. He had a slightly elevated ALAT of 86 U/l with normal ASAT and LDH; other liver-dependent measurements were normal, but his gamma glutamyl transferase (GGT) was slightly elevated (54 U/l). His fasting plasma glucose, thyroid function, and kreatinine concentration were all normal. Finally, the apoE genotype was E3/E3.

The diagnosis

When the presenting lipid phenotype is a combined or mixed hyperlipidemia, secondary causes of dyslipidemia should be ruled out. First of all diabetic dyslipidemia should be eliminated and a fasting glucose sample is sufficient to rule this out. The intake of excessive amounts of alcohol should also be ruled out since this may result in elevated triglycerides. Typically, HDL-cholesterol is disproportionately elevated in alcohol-induced hypertriglyceridemia. In some women, estrogen use may cause the same disturbances (high triglycerides with elevated HDL-cholesterol). Otherwise, high triglycerides are always accompanied by decreased HDL-cholesterol. Tests for thyroid function, renal function, and liver function should be carried out. If these are all negative a primary type of hyperlipidemia should be considered. The family history is of paramount importance and should be recorded in detail. A fasting lipid profile of first degree relatives is certainly helpful. This may be done by the GP of each relative or by the Lipid Clinic. The most likely differential diagnosis in the case of primary combined hyperlipidemia is shown in Table 1: familial combined hyperlipidemia (FCHL), familial hypertriglyceridemia (FHTG), and familial dysbetalipoproteinemia (FD).

FCHL is typified by a positive family history for premature atherosclerosis, high apoB concentrations (usually above 1.2 g/l), and multiple lipid phenotypes in first degree relatives (see also type 1). Usually FCHL patients are insulin resistant and around 80% may have the metabolic syndrome.

The most likely diagnosis in our patient is FCHL, although exact data on the lipid profile of first degree relatives are lacking.

FCHL: the background

Familial combined hyperlipidemia (FCHL) is the most frequent familial dyslipidemia resulting in premature atherosclerosis.[1-5] Several reports have suggested that FCHL is a monogenic disorder with different modifying genes.[6-8] The gene directly responsible for FCHL has not been identified yet, although several candidates have been described.[9,10] A recently identified gene on chromosome 11, the apolipoprotein (apo) AV gene, seems to be one of the most promising candidates due to its strong effects on fasting plasma triglyceride concentrations in FCHL.[11] In addition, much attention has been drawn to the upstream stimulatory factor (USF proteins) located within the chromosome 1q21–23.[12,13] Finally, several authors now believe that different genes may be involved in the expression of the phenotype of FCHL.[7,9,10,14]

The diagnosis of FCHL is based on clinical criteria such as the presence of 'multiple type hyperlipidemia',[1-5] a positive family history of premature

86

Table 1 Differential diagnosis for inherited types of combined hyperlipidemia

Parameter	FCHL	FHTG	FD	Autosomal dominant FD
Lipid profile	Mildly elevated cholesterol, low HDL-cholesterol, mildly elevated triglycerides	Mildly elevated cholesterol, 3× elevated triglycerides, low HDL-cholesterol	Mildly elevated cholesterol, low HDL-cholesterol, mildly elevated triglycerides	Mildly elevated cholesterol, low HDL-cholesterol, mildly elevated triglycerides
apoB	>1.2 g/l	0.6–0.9 g/l	0.6–0.9 g/l	0.6–0.9 g/l
Mode of inheritance	Dominant	Dominant	Recessive in classical forms where homozygosity for apoE2 is necessary	Dominant
apoE genotype	E3 or E4	E3 or E4	Always homozygous for E2	Mutated apoE (for example, E3 Leiden)
Atherogenicity	++	+/−	++	+
Treatment (lifestyle intervention in all cases)	Statins +/− fibrates and/or cholesterol absorption inhibitor	Fibrates (resins contraindicated due to triglycerides elevation)	Statins or fibrates	Statins or fibrates
Pancreatitis	+/−	+	+/−	+/−
Lipid phenotype in first degree relatives	Multiple types	Only hypertriglyceridemia	Usually normal in heterozygotes for apoE2	Usually combined hyperlipidemia in heterozygotes for mutated apoE

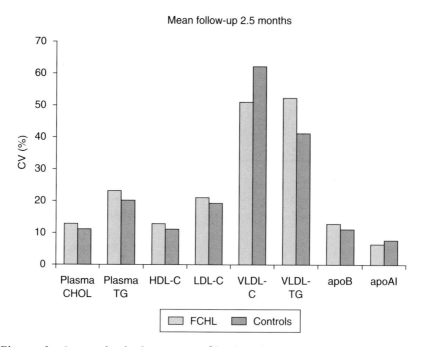

Figure 1 *Inter-individual variations of lipids and lipoproteins in healthy subjects and in untreated patients with FCHL. CHOL, cholesterol; TG, triglycerides; CV, coefficient of variation. Modified from Delawi D et al. Clin Chim Acta 2003; 328: 139–45 with permission from Elsevier.*

coronary heart disease (CHD), and increased plasma apoB, reflecting VLDL overproduction.[15,16] Originally multiple type hyperlipidemia meant both, different phenotypes in one pedigree at the time and changing phenotypes in one subject throughout time.[5] The latter has been challenged recently and when compared to healthy subjects, the intra-individual lipoprotein variability seems to be similar in FCHL subjects (Figure 1). Other metabolic characteristics in FCHL are, among others, impaired chylomicron remnant clearance,[17,18] high levels of small dense LDL,[19] the presence of insulin resistance,[20,21] disturbed postprandial free fatty acid (FFA) metabolism,[20,22,23] and impaired FFA uptake by fibroblasts and adipocytes,[24] resulting in enhanced FFA flux to the liver[20,22] (Box 1). Finally, decreased *in vitro* activity of hormone sensitive lipase has been described in Swedish FCHL patients,[24] but not in Finnish patients,[25] or in Dutch patients based on *in vivo* studies.[26]

Based on the metabolic abnormalities described in FCHL,[27] several investigators have attempted to reach consensus on the clinical identification of the FCHL phenotype.[28] It was concluded that the hyperTG-hyperapoB was the

---

Box 1   Familial combined hyperlipidemia (FCHL): metabolic and clinical characteristics

---

- Fasting combined hyperlipidemia usually with low HDL-cholesterol
- VLDL overproduction
- Elevated fasting apoB
- Decreased chylomicron remnant clearance
- Postprandial elevated free fatty acids (FFA)
- Postprandially increased ketone bodies reflecting enhanced hepatic FFA flux
- Decreased hormone sensitive activity in a subset of patients
- Small dense LDL
- Insulin resistance
- Decreased action of acylation stimulating protein (ASP) (*in vitro*)
- High fasting complement component 3 (C3)
- Impaired postprandial C3 response
- Insufficient response to therapy
- Enhanced margination of apoB *in vivo*

---

most characteristic presentation of patients with FCHL. This approach is justified because several metabolic disorders linked to different genes may ultimately lead to the same phenotype of hepatic apoB overproduction and fasting dyslipidemia. The proposed definition will help to identify patients with the FCHL phenotype in clinical practice, as long as the genetic marker for the disease has not been found. It should also be stressed that dyslipidemia in FCHL is only modest in contrast to, for example, familial hypercholesterolemia (FH) with strikingly elevated LDL-cholesterol levels (Figure 2).

Since FCHL and the metabolic syndrome share so many clinical characteristics and metabolic disturbances,[5,20,21] it has always been difficult to separate the two disorders. One of the striking differences may be the mode of inheritance and the effect of environmental factors on the expression of both phenotypes. While in FCHL a clear dominant inheritance pattern is observed, with the environment as important modifier, the influence of diet and lifestyle has a more potent impact in the metabolic syndrome. For example, dietary interventions and lifestyle modifications may be sufficient to correct several metabolic abnormalities in the metabolic syndrome,[29] while drug treatment is almost always necessary in FCHL.[5] Furthermore, the prevalence of the metabolic syndrome is much higher than the predicted prevalence of FCHL.[30] Finally, derangements of carbohydrate metabolism seem to play a more important role in the expression of the metabolic

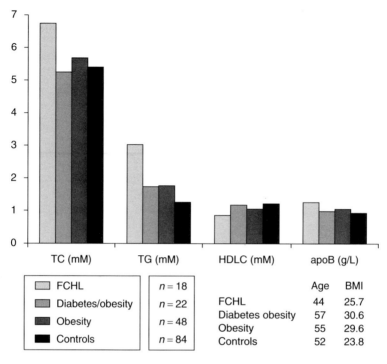

Figure 2 *Comparison of fasting lipid profile in FCHL and other conditions associated with hyperlipidemia in comparison to healthy subjects. Fasting plasma lipids are only marginally elevated in FCHL subjects.*

syndrome than in FCHL and plasma apoB levels in FCHL are not fully associated with insulin resistance.[31]

FCHL: the treatment

The initial treatment in FCHL is lifestyle intervention with a diet rich in mono- and polyunsaturated fatty acids ('lots of olive oil and fish'), calory restriction, and weight reduction. Everybody should be advised to exercise, since this leads to improved insulin sensitivity, lipid and glucose profiles, and blood pressure. Special attention should be directed to reducing the waist circumference. Smoking should be discouraged.

   In the case of FCHL, lifestyle interventions are usually not sufficient and lipid-lowering therapy should be initiated. Statins are the drug of choice in FCHL. They reduce hepatic apoB secretion (which is the major metabolic disturbance in

FCHL), improve postprandial lipemia,[32–34] and may even lead to improved fatty acid metabolism.[34,35] However, even combination therapy with fibrates does not always lead to normalization of the lipid profile in FCHL.[18] The use of insulin sensitizers like the glitazones seems reasonable but has not been studied in detail in FCHL, in contrast to extensive experience in diabetes which shares many metabolic disturbances with FCHL.[36] Finally, novel developments will lead to new therapeutic approaches directed not only to improvement of the lipoprotein profile but also to amelioration of the chronic inflammatory situation associated with FCHL.[37]

References

1. Goldstein JL, Schrott HG, Hazzard WR, Bierman EL, Motulsky AG. Hyperlipidemia in coronary heart disease. II. Genetic analysis of lipid levels in 176 families and delineation of a new inherited disorder, combined hyperlipidemia. J Clin Invest 1973; 52: 1544–68.

2. Nikkila EA, Aro A. Family study of sperum lipids and lipoproteins in coronary heart-disease. Lancet 1973; 1: 954–9.

3. Rose HG, Kranz P, Weinstock M, Juliano J, Haft JI. Inheritance of combined hyperlipoproteinemia: evidence for a new lipoprotein phenotype. Am J Med 1973; 54(2): 148–60.

4. Pitkanen OP, Nuutila P, Raitakari OT et al. Coronary flow reserve in young men with familial combined hyperlipidemia. Circulation 1999; 99(13): 1678–84.

5. Castro Cabezas M, de Bruin TW, Erkelens DW. Familial combined hyperlipidemia:1973–1991. Neth J Med 1992; 40(1–2): 83–95.

6. Aouizerat BE, Allayee H, Bodnar J et al. Novel genes for familial combined hyper-lipidemia. Curr Opin Lipidol 1999; 10(2); 113–22.

7. Aouizerat BE, Allayee H, Cantor RM et al. A genome scan for familial combined hyperlipidemia reveals evidence of linkage with a locus on chromosome 11. Am J Hum Genet 1999; 65(2): 397–412.

8. Pajukanta P, Terwilliger JD, Perola M et al. Genomewide scan for familial combined hyperlipidemia genes in Finnish families, suggesting multiple susceptibility loci influencing triglyceride, cholesterol, and apolipoprotein B levels. Am J Hum Genet 1999; 64(5): 1453–63.

9. Jarvik GP, Brunzell JD, Austin MA et al. Genetic predictors of FCHL in four large pedigrees. Influence of ApoB level major locus predicted genotype and LDL subclass phenotype. Arterioscler Thromb 1994; 14(11): 1687–94.

10. Ribalta J, La Ville AE, Vallve JC et al. A variation in the apolipoprotein C-III gene is associated with an increased number of circulating VLDL and IDL particles in familial combined hyperlipidemia. J Lipid Res 1997; 38(6): 1061–9.

11. Ribalta J, Figuera L, Fernandez-Ballart J et al. Newly identified apolipoprotein AV gene predisposes to high plasma triglycerides in familial combined hyperlipidemia. Clin Chem 2002; 48(9): 1597–600.

12. Shoulders CC, Naoumova RP. USF1 implicated in the aetiology of familial combined hyperlipidemia and the metabolic syndrome. Trends Mol Med 2004; 10: 362–5.

13. Wang X, Gargalovic P, Wong J et al. Hyplip2, a new gene for combined hyperlipidemia and increased atherosclerosis. Arterioscl Thromb Vasc Biol 2004; 24: 1–7.

14. Badzioch MD, Igo RP, Gagnon F et al. Low-density lipoprotein particle size loci in familial combined hyperlipidemia. Evidence for multiple loci from a genome scan. Arterioscl Thromb Vasc Biol 2004; 24: 1–9.

15. Chait A, Albers JJ, and Brunzell JD. Very low density lipoprotein overproduction in genetic forms of hypertriglyceridaemia. Eur J Clin Invest 1980; 10(1): 17–22.

16. Janus ED, Nicoll AM, Turner PR, Magill P, and Lewis B. Kinetic bases of the primary hyperlipidaemias: studies of apolipoprotein B turnover in genetically defined subjects. Eur J Clin Invest 1980; 10(2 Pt 1): 161–72.

17. Castro Cabezas M, de Bruin TWA, Jansen H et al. Impaired chylomicron remnant clearance in familial combined hyperlipidemia. Arterioscler Thromb 1993; 13: 804–14.

18. Castro Cabezas M, de Bruin TWA, Kock LAW et al. Postprandial apolipoprotein B100 and apo B48 in Familial Combined Hyperlipidemia before and after reduction of fasting plasma triglycerides. Eur J Clin Invest 1994; 24: 669–78.

19. Austin MA, Brunzell JD, Fitch WL, Krauss RM. Inheritance of low density lipoprotein subclass patterns in familial combined hyperlipidemia. Arteriosclerosis 1990; 10(4): 520–30.

20. Castro Cabezas M, de Bruin TWA, de Valk HW et al. Impaired fatty acid metabolism in familial combined hyperlipidemia. A mechanism associating hepatic apolipoprotein B overproduction and insulin resistance. J Clin Invest 1993; 92: 160–8.

21. Ascaso JF, Merchante A, Lorente RI et al. A study of insulin resistance using the minimal model in nondiabetic familial combined hyperlipidemic patients. Metabolism 1998; 47(5): 508–13.

22. Meijssen S, van Dijk H, Verseyden C, Erkelens DW, Castro Cabezas M. Delayed and exaggerated postprandial complement 3 response in familial combined hyperlipidemia. Arterioscl Thromb Vasc Biol 2002; 22: 811–16.

23. Sniderman AD, Cianflone K, Arner P, Summers LK, Frayn KN. The adipocyte, fatty acid trapping, and atherogenesis, Arterioscler Thromb Vasc Biol 1998; 18(2): 147–51.

24. Reynisdottir S, Eriksson M, Angelin B, Arner P. Impaired activation of adipocyte lipolysis in familial combined hyperlipidemia. J Clin Invest 1995; 95(5): 2161–9.

25. Ylitalo K, Large V, Pajukanta P et al. Reduced hormone-sensitive lipase activity is not a major metabolic defect in Finnish FCHL families. Atherosclerosis 2000; 153(2): 373–81.

26. Meijssen S, Derksen RJ, Bilecen S, Erkelens DW, Castro Cabezas M. In vivo modulation of plasma free fatty acids in patients with familial combined hyperlipidemia using lipid-lowering medication. J Clin Endocrinol Metab 2002; 87: 1576–80.

27. Sniderman AD, Ribalta J, Castro Cabezas M. How should FCHL be defined and how should we think about its metabolic bases? Nutr Metab Cardiovasc Dis 2001; 11(4): 259–73 [Erratum in: Nutr Metab Cardiovasc Dis 2001; 11(6): 412].

28. Sniderman AD, Castro Cabezas M, Ribalta J et al. A Proposal to redefine familial combined hyperlipidemia – third workshop on FCHL held in Barcelona from 3 to 5 May 2001, during the scientific sessions of the European Society for Clinical Investigation. Eur J Clin Invest 2002; 32(2): 71–3.

29. Knowler WC, Barrett-Connor E, Fowler SE et al. Reduction in the incidence of type 2 diabetes with lifestyle intervention or metformin. N Engl J Med 2002; 346(6): 393–403.

30. Park YW, Zhu S, Palaniappan L et al. The metabolic syndrome: prevalence and associated risk factor findings in the US population from the Third National Health and Nutrition Examination Survey, 1988–1994. Arch Intern Med 2003; 163(4): 427–36.

31. Purnell JQ, Kahn SE, Schwartz RS, Brunzell JD. Relationship of insulin sensitivity and ApoB levels to intra-abdominal fat in subjects with familial combined hyperlipidemia. Arterioscler Thromb Vasc Biol 2001; 21(4): 567–72.

32. Castro Cabezas M, de Bruin TWA, Kock LAW et al. Simvastatin improves chylomicron remnant removal in familial combined hyperlipidemia without changing chylomicron conversion. Metabolism 1993; 42: 497–503.

33. Castro Cabezas M, de Bruin TWA, Jansen H et al. Impaired chylomicron remnant clearance in familial combined hyperlipidemia. Arterioscler Thromb 1993; 13: 804–14.

34. Castro Cabezas M, Verseyden C, Jansen H, Meijssen S. Effects of atorvastatin on the clearance of triglyceride rich lipoproteins in familial combined hyperlipidemia. J Clin Endocrinol Metab 2004; 89: 5972–80.

35. Halkes CJM, van Dijk H, De Jaegere PPTh et al. Postprandial increase of complement component 3 in normolipidemic patients with coronary artery disease. Effects of expanded dose simvastatin. Arterioscl Thromb Vasc Biol 2001; 21: 1526–30.

36. Van Wijk JPH, Castro Cabezas M, de Koning EJP, Rabelink TJ. Rosiglitazone improves postprandial triglyceride and free fatty acid metabolism in type 2 diabetes. Diabetes Care 2005; 28: 844–9.

37. Van Oostrom AJHHM, Van Wijk JPH, Castro Cabezas M. Lipaemia, inflammation and atherosclerosis: novel opportunities in the understanding and treatment of atherosclerosis. Drugs 2004; 64 (Suppl 2): 19–41.

93

Case 19

MANAGEMENT OF COMBINED
HYPERLIPIDEMIA

Philip J Barter

Patient profile

Peter is a 42-year-old man who had had three myocardial infarctions at ages 29, 32, and 33 years. His myocardial function was so compromised after the last episode that he was considered for a heart transplant, which was performed at age 34 years. He had a lipid abnormality for which he had been receiving treatment with a statin. After the transplant, statin therapy was stopped because of a concern that the cyclosporin he was taking to prevent organ rejection may interact adversely with the statin. He was referred to the Lipid Clinic in December 1997, 4 months after the transplant. His plasma lipids at this time were: LDL-cholesterol 9.6 mmol/l, HDL-cholesterol 0.6 mmol/l, and triglyceride 5.7 mmol/l.

A family history of premature coronary heart disease (CHD) and dyslipidemia suggested that he had familial combined hyperlipidemia.

It was decided that the risk of a future coronary event was so high that it was essential to re-introduce therapy to control Peter's plasma lipids. Atorvastatin was re-introduced and titrated up to a dose of 80 mg/day. His creatine kinase (CK) level remained normal. His plasma lipids measured 3 months after re-starting on atorvastatin were: LDL-cholesterol 5.5 mmol/l, HDL-cholesterol 0.7 mmol/l, and triglyceride 3.5 mmol/l.

The atorvastatin dose was reduced to 40 mg/day and gemfibrozil was added, initially at a dose of 600 mg/day, increasing after 1 month to 600 mg twice daily. Two months after commencing this combination, his CK level remained normal but the lipid profile was still undesirable: LDL-cholesterol 4.8 mmol/l, HDL-cholesterol 0.9 mmol/l, and triglyceride 2.6 mmol/l.

Niacin was then added at increasing doses to a final level of 3 g/day and cholestyramine was introduced at a dose of 8 g/day.

After 12 months on this combination of drugs Peter's plasma lipids were: LDL-cholesterol 2.8 mmol/l, HDL-cholesterol 1.2 mmol/l, and triglyceride 1.4 mmol/l.

His CK level remained normal despite the combination of lipid-lowering drugs being taken with cyclosporin. His cardiac function was excellent, and he had been back at work for 8 months.

As an intelligent man who understood clearly potentially major benefits of maintaining this lipid profile, Peter's adherence to the medication was excellent, despite periodic unpleasant flushing and itching associated with the niacin.

One month later (after 13 months on combination therapy), Peter developed severe muscle pain and was found to have a CK level more than 30 times above the upper limit of normal. Four days earlier he had visited his primary care physician with an upper respiratory tract infection, for which he had been prescribed erythromycin. The erythromycin and all lipid-lowering medication were stopped. The muscle pain rapidly subsided and his CK level fell, returning to normal 2 weeks after all therapy had stopped. He now felt well.

After another 2 weeks, it was decided to slowly reintroduce lipid-lowering therapy. Eight weeks later, Peter was back on the full combination of drugs and his lipid levels were again under good control. His CK level remained normal.

When seen, 2 years after the episode of myositis, Peter was still on the full combination of lipid-lowering drugs plus cyclosporin. He felt well and his cardiac function remained excellent.

He continues to feel well, with excellent cardiac function. The only change to his lipid-lowering therapy has been to replace cholestyramine with the cholesterol absorption inhibitor, ezetimibe.

Issues

This case raises several issues.

- It is possible to correct even the most severe lipid abnormalities in most people by using combinations of lipid-modifying drugs.
- Combinations do increase the risk of myopathy, although in patients with severe combined hyperlipidemia, the potential benefits probably greatly outweigh the risk.
- It is essential to know which drugs may interact adversely with lipid-lowering agents and to make sure that the patient also has this knowledge.
- Macrolide antibiotics such as erythromycin are especially dangerous when given with a statin and are well known to increase greatly the risk of statin-induced myositis.
- Adherence to combination medication is helped if the patient truly understands both the potential benefits as well as the potential risks.

Combinations of statins and fibrates

The combination of statins and fibrates has a clear superiority over monotherapy with either class of agent in people with severe combined hyperlipidemia. Overall, the statin–fibrate combination is well tolerated, although the combination is known to be associated with an increased risk of myopathy. While the absolute risk of myopathy is low with the combination of most statins with most fibrates,[1] it is increased substantially when the fibrate is gemfibrozil and the statin is cerivastatin. This latter observation contributed to the decision to withdraw cerivastatin from the market. In contrast to the effects of gemfibrozil, when fenofibrate is combined with a statin the risk of myopathy appears to be no different from that observed with the statin alone. The potential clinical benefits of combining a statin and a fibrate are greatest in people in whom the dyslipidemia is a component of type 2 diabetes, insulin resistance, or the metabolic syndrome. In such people fibrates (unlike statins) have major cardioprotective benefits beyond those predicted by the changes in plasma lipid concentration. In other words, in people whose dyslipidemia is associated with type 2 diabetes, insulin resistance or the metabolic syndrome,[2] it seems that the two classes of drug may reduce cardiovascular risk by different mechanisms. Circumstantial evidence strongly supports the use of a statin–fibrate combination to reduce cardiovascular risk in such people.

Combinations of statins and niacin

The combination of a statin with niacin is another effective approach to improve the lipid profile in patients with combined hyperlipidemia. Furthermore, the statin–niacin combination has been shown to result in a substantial reduction in both atherosclerosis progression and cardiovascular events.[3] The flushing and itching associated with earlier formulations of niacin are much less with niaspan, an extended-release form of the drug, which is much better tolerated by most patients.

Combinations of statins and ezetimibe

To achieve recommended LDL-cholesterol targets in patients with high levels, it is often necessary to combine a statin with an additional LDL-lowering agent; ideally this should be the cholesterol absorption inhibitor, ezetimibe.

97

Conclusion

Much current attention is paid to the adverse effects of statins, especially when given in combination with fibrates. However, it is worth considering the potential benefits relative to risk of such a combination before deciding to abandon it completely. It is perhaps worth asking: should a high-risk patient with combined hyperlipidemia be denied a combination that may reduce risk of a future coronary event by 50% or more because of a risk of severe myopathy that is probably of the order of about 0.1%?

So, if monotherapy with a statin does not correct the lipid profile in high-risk people with combined hyperlipidemia, seriously consider adding ezetimibe to maximize the LDL-cholesterol lowering and either fenofibrate or niaspan (or both) to maximize the reduction in triglyceride and the increase in HDL-cholesterol.

References

1. Shanahan RL, Kerzee JA, Sandhoff BG, Carroll NM, Merenich JA. Low myopathy rates associated with statins as monotherapy or combination therapy with interacting drugs in a group model health maintenance organization. Pharmacotherapy 2005; 25: 345–51.
2. Steiner G. Fibrates in the metabolic syndrome and in diabetes. Endocrinol Metab Clin North Am 2004; 33: 545–55.
3. Brown BG, Zhao XQ, Chait A et al. Simvastatin and niacin, antioxidant vitamins, or the combination for the prevention of coronary disease. N Engl J Med 2001; 345: 1583–92.

Case 20

FAT IN THE LIVER: A FEATURE OF INSULIN RESISTANCE, DYSLIPIDEMIA, AND ATHEROSCLEROSIS?

Dirk Müller-Wieland

A 47-year-old man (BJ) came to my office, because his brother had suffered from a myocardial infarction at the age of 54. The cardiologist recommended his brother to lower LDL-cholesterol levels below 70 mg/dl, because he was overweight, and had low HDL-cholesterol levels and clinically overt type 2 diabetes. BJ did not remember his father's clinical history because his parents were divorced when he was a child. His mother, however, suffered like his brother from type 2 diabetes. He did not smoke, apparently took two to three drinks per week, and there was no history of any other clinically relevant disease.

The physical examination showed a healthy appearing male individuum with a height of 178 cm, a waist circumference of 108 cm, and blood pressure of 125/80 mm Hg. The laboratory investigation revealed a dyslipidemia (triglycerides 210 mg/dl, HDL-cholesterol 38 mg/dl, LDL-cholesterol 120 mg/dl, and total cholesterol 200 mg/dl). Fasting glucose was 102 mg/dl and an oral glucose tolerance test revealed overt type 2 diabetes, i.e. a 2-hour glucose value of 265 mg/dl. This test was repeated after 2 weeks and confirmed the diagnosis. Other parameters of clinical chemistry showed no evidence of microalbuminuria; however, liver enzymes were slightly elevated (GOT 40 mU/l, GPT 20, γGT 40, cholinesterase 8000 U), but ferritin levels and autoimmune as well as viral parameters for the differential diagnosis of inflammatory liver disease were negative. Ultrasound investigation of the upper abdomen showed a slightly enlarged liver with diffuse homogeneous hyperdense findings corresponding to the ultrasound phenomenon called 'bright liver'.

Taken together, a type 2 diabetes was diagnosed in this patient, presented by dyslipidemia with evidence of nonalcoholic fatty liver disease. As initial treatment the patient was recommended to take a hypocaloric Mediterranean diet and to increase his physical activity for at least 30 minutes per day. After about 4 months the patient reduced his weight by 7 kg and his blood sugar levels were normalized, i.e. in the fasting state below 100 mg/dl, and the lipid levels improved (cholesterol 175 mg/dl, triglyceride 170 mg/dl, LDL-cholesterol 101 mg/dl, HDL-cholesterol 40 mg/dl). The echogenicity of the liver decreased significantly and the hepatic enzyme levels were normalized.

Commentary

This 'simple' case shows that family members of patients with coronary heart disease (CHD) should be screened for features of the metabolic syndrome, such as screening for overt type 2 diabetes or glucose intolerance, dyslipidemia and increased waist circumference. Therefore, I intend to catch your attention and interest, because this is an example of the typical 'undercover' patient who presents with no complaints, believes that he is healthy, but in fact is a 'cardiovascular time bomb' considering his positive family history of early CHD, features of the metabolic syndrome, and type 2 diabetes.

In addition, the clinical phenomenon on which I would like to focus in this context is biochemical and clinical evidence of nonalcoholic fatty liver disease in this patient, which was greatly improved by weight loss induced by diet and increased physical activity. Reversal of nonalcoholic fatty liver disease by moderate weight reduction in patients with type 2 diabetes has recently been described and investigated in greater detail by Petersen et al.[1] They investigated whether moderate weight reduction in patients with type 2 diabetes decreases intrahepatic lipid content as determined by ^{1}H magnetic resonance spectroscopy, and whether this might be related to improvement of blood glucose levels and hepatic insulin resistance. They showed that reduction of intrahepatic lipid content was associated with improvement in basal and insulin-stimulated hepatic glucose metabolism, suggesting that moderate weight loss can normalize fasting hyperglycemia in patients with type 2 diabetes by mobilizing a relatively small pool of intrahepatic lipids, which is associated with a reversal of hepatic insulin resistance and normalization of basal glucose production rates. This adds to a growing body of clinical and molecular evidence that increased fat content in non-adipose tissue, also called 'ectopic' lipid accumulation, is associated with insulin resistance. In particular, increased lipid content in liver is associated with the metabolic syndrome and type 2 diabetes (see Box 1).[2–4]

What did I learn?

'Ectopic' lipid accumulation might be a novel mechanism of insulin resistance. Several cell and animal studies and an increasing number of clinical studies

100

Box 1   NAFLD: a feature of the metabolic syndrome

- Prevalence
  - c. 35% in the general population (75% in obese and 15% in nonobese)
  - 25% in individuals with normal fasting glucose
  - 45% in individuals with impaired fasting glucose
  - 60% in newly diagnosed diabetics
  - 90% of individuals with NAFLD have type 2 diabetes or one feature of the metabolic syndrome

- NAFLD increases the risk for cirrhosis and there is a higher prevalence of HCV antibodies in patients with type 2 diabetes
- Increased risk for NASH and hepatocellular carcinoma
- Ultrasound for diagnosing steatosis with a degree > 33%:
  sensitivity 60–94%
  specificity 88–95%
- Reduction of steatosis, which is associated with improved insulin sensitivity by weight reduction and drugs, such as metformin as well as rosiglitazone and pioglitazone

NAFLD, nonalcoholic fatty liver disease; NASH, nonalcoholic steatohepatitis; MS, metabolic syndrome. For further details, see text and reviews.[2–4]

---

support the hypothesis of Unger[5] and McGarry[6] that an increased intracellular lipid accumulation in nonfat cells is associated with a disturbance of the respective functions, i.e. insulin resistance in the case of insulin action. Thereby ectopic lipid accumulation in liver but also in skeletal muscle might be a mechanism that brings new light to the interaction between body weight and insulin sensitivity. If it is not the amount of subcutaneous fat but rather the amount of ectopic fat accumulation that determines insulin resistance, one would predict that isolated removal of subcutaneous fat would have no effect on insulin sensitivity. This question was recently answered by an elegant clinical study by Klein et al.,[7] in which they investigated the effect of liposuction in obese women with either normal glucose tolerance or type 2 diabetes. The volume of subcutaneous fat was reduced in those groups by approximately 10 kg. Insulin sensitivity of liver, skeletal muscle, and adipose tissue were evaluated before and 10–12 weeks after abdominal liposuction. The intervention had no significant effect on the insulin sensitivity of these tissues and other features of the metabolic syndrome, such as blood pressure or plasma lipids. Furthermore, inflammatory markers in plasma such as C-reactive protein, interleukin-6 and TNF-α were also not changed. Donnelly et al.[8] have recently shown, using orally fat stable isotopes and medically indicated liver biopsies in patients with nonalcoholic fatty liver disease, that almost 60% of triglycerides in liver derive from non-esterified fatty acids (NEFA), about 25% from *de novo* lipogenesis, and about 15% from the diet. The *de novo* lipogenesis was elevated in the fasting state, indicating that both elevated peripheral fatty acids and *de novo* lipogenesis contribute to the accumulation of hepatic fat in nonalcoholic fatty liver disease.

How much did this case alter my clinical practice?

The concept of ectopic lipid accumulation might be an answer to many basic unresolved clinical observations, for example, that insulin sensitivity does not correlate with the amount of subcutaneous fat, that insulin sensitivity is greatly increased by only a modest body weight reduction of only 5–10%, and that not all obese individuals are insulin resistant. Taken together the metabolic syndrome represents a group of clinical disorders related not only to insulin resistance but perhaps rather to altered liporegulation or 'lipid spillover' (reviewed in Unger[5] and McGarry[6]). Therefore, it is interesting to note that some insulin sensitivity treatment strategies, like weight reduction, glitazones, and metformin can reduce hepatic fat content. Anti-diabetic agents acting to improve insulin sensitivity might perhaps be also better understood as 'anti-lipotoxic' drugs.

The liver comes into focus. The liver is an essential organ for the production and catabolism of lipoproteins, glucose metabolism, and therefore features of insulin resistance. Furthermore, the liver plays an essential role in determining inflammatory reactions. Considering all this evidence together, the liver appears to be a key player not only in the development and treatment of the metabolic syndrome, but also of the associated cardiovascular risk induced by atherosclerosis.

References

1. Petersen KF, Dufour S, Befroy D et al. Reversal of nonalcoholic hepatic steatosis, hepatic insulin resistance, and hyperglycemia by moderate weight reduction in patients with type 2 diabetes. Diabetes 2005; 54: 603–8.
2. Adams LA, Angulot P. Recent concepts in non-alcoholic fatty liver disease. Diabetic. Med 2005; 22: 1129–33.
3. Tolman KG, Fonseca V, Tan MH, Dalpiaz A. Narrative review: hepatobiliary disease in type 2 diabetes mellitus. Ann Intern Med 2004; 141: 946–56.

4. Medina J, Garcia-Buey L, Fernandez-Salazar LI, Moreno-Otero R. Approach to the pathogenesis and treatment of nonalcoholic steatohepatitis. Diabetes Care 2004; 27: 2057–66.
5. Unger RH. Minireview: weapons of lean body mass destruction: the role of ectopic lipids in the metabolic syndrome. Endocrinology 2003; 144: 5159–65.
6. McGarry JD. Dysregulation of fatty acid metabolism in the etiology of type 2 diabetes. Diabetes 2002; 51: 7–18.
7. Klein S, Fontana L, Young L et al. Absence of an effect of liposuction on insulin action and risk factors for coronary heart disease. N Engl J Med 2004; 350: 2549–57.
8. Donnelly KL, Smith CI, Schwarzenberg SJ et al. Sources of fatty acids stored in liver and secreted via lipoproteins in patients with nonalcoholic fatty liver disease. J Clin Invest 2005; 115: 1343–51.

Case 21

MIXED LIPEMIA WITH STRIKING PHYSICAL SIGNS

D John Betteridge

Case history

A Caucasian man presented to the Lipid Clinic following the finding of severe mixed lipemia at the age of 60 years. Of importance in the past history his lipid profile was first assessed when he was 32 years old because of the family history. His brother had developed nodules over both elbows and was found to be dyslipidemic. The patient also recalled that his brother had nodules on the palms of his hands. At the time of diagnosis this patient also had small nodules on his elbows.

He was prescribed Atromid (clofibrate) which he took for approximately 9 years. The nodules disappeared. There are no records of his plasma lipids at that time. He then stopped the drug because he developed gallstones and required cholecystectomy.

He presented again at the age of 60 years for an opinion on his dyslipidemia following the development of heart disease in his brother, who had developed angina which required coronary artery bypass surgery. Some 5 years previously the brother had undergone surgery for an abdominal aortic aneurysm.

He was a nonsmoker and did not drink excess alcohol. He had no symptoms referable to the cardiovascular system. His diet was good and he had followed a low-fat diet since his thirties. There were no stigmata of hyperlipidemia. Blood pressure was 114/73 mm Hg. His lipid profile showed severe mixed lipemia with total cholesterol of 11.5 mmol/l and triglycerides of 9.08 mmol/l. There is no record of apoprotein B on this occasion but lipoprotein (a) was raised at 0.77 g/l. HDL-cholesterol was 0.89 mmol/l. Thyroid function was normal and plasma glucose was 5.2 mmol/l. Liver and renal function were normal.

He was started on combination therapy with atorvastatin 10 mg/day and bezafibrate 400 mg/day in the form of the sustained-release preparation.

Some 3 months later he came to our clinic for further assessment. By this time there had been a substantial improvement in the lipid profile. His cholesterol had fallen to 4.1 mmol/l and triglycerides to 1.97 mmol/l. Hepatic and renal function were normal, as was the creatine phosphokinase. He did not complain of any side effects from the drugs, in particular there was no muscle pain. On this occasion he complained of some atypical chest pain but a thallium stress test was completely normal.

Because of the nature of the dyslipidemia and the history suggestive of xanthomata, his apoprotein E phenotype was assessed and found to be 2/2, confirming the clinical diagnosis of type III hyperlipoproteinemia. When last seen he was taking the same medication with a cholesterol of 3.7 mmol/l, triglycerides of 2.57 mmol/l, HDL-cholesterol 1.4 mmol/l, and calculated LDL-cholesterol of 1.1 mmol/l. Hepatic function was normal apart from a borderline gamma glutamyl transferase at 50, which was not thought to be of clinical significance.

Learning points

Type III hyperlipoproteinemia. Biochemistry and pathogenesis. This is a rare but very interesting condition. It has several synonyms based on some of the defining laboratory characteristics used to make the diagnosis over the last four decades: broad beta disease, dysbetalipoproteinemia, floating beta disease, and remnant particle disease. It represents an interesting interaction between genetic factors and acquired conditions. It has provided evidence of the atherogenicity of remnant particles that is of relevance to other dyslipidemias such as those that accompany type 2 diabetes, the metabolic syndrome, and chronic kidney disease. In addition, it has become apparent that apoprotein E isoforms not only underlie the basis of type 3 disease but also contribute to the variance of plasma cholesterol concentrations in the general population.

Clinical biochemistry demonstrates elevated plasma cholesterol and triglycerides of roughly equivalent degree and in addition there are classical findings on lipoprotein electrophoresis and ultracentrifugation, which reflects the accumulation of remnants of chylomicron and very low density lipoprotein (VLDL) metabolism, namely β-VLDL. On lipoprotein electrophoresis there is a characteristic broad beta band and on ultra centrifugation the VLDL fraction has a cholesterol to triglyceride molar ratio >0.6 (floating beta lipoproteins). These investigations can be performed in specialist centers; however, nowadays it is generally simpler to obtain apoprotein E phenotypes in suspected cases.

Almost all cases are heterozygous for apoprotein E2. Two-thirds of individuals are homozygous for E3, which is the normal allele, whereas only 1% are homozygous for E2. Apoprotein E2 has a cysteine residue instead of the normal arginine at position 158. This substitution is associated with reduced ability of the apoprotein to bind to the LDL receptor (Apo-B, apo-E receptor).

Although apoprotein E2 homozygosity is relatively common, type III disease is rare at approximately 1:5000 to 1:10 000. Therefore it is necessary for another factor to be present for the syndrome to develop. Other abnormalities are needed to 'stress' the remnant particle removal system for these particles to accumulate, such as familial combined hyperlipidemia, familial hypertriglyceridemia, and familial hypercholesterolemia. Environmental factors can also interact to produce the syndrome such as obesity, type 2 diabetes, and hypothyroidism.

Type III disease is generally inherited as an autosomal recessive trait with variable penetrance, but rare variants of apoprotein E involving substitution of acidic or neutral amino acids for basic ones in the receptor-binding region can be inherited as a dominant trait. The presence of these substitutions (e.g. arginine 142-cysteine; lysine146-glutamic acid) are sufficient for development of the type III phenotype, although it can be exacerbated by other genetic and environmental factors. It is likely that these mutations affect the binding of remnants to the receptor. Apoprotein E Leiden, which is characterized by a tandem duplication of amino acid residues 121–127 of apoprotein E, probably leads to a conformational change in the receptor-binding region.

Cinical features. This rare condition is more prevalent in men than women and affected women are usually postmenopausal. There have been reports of amelioration of the disease in women following hormone replacement therapy.

The xanthomata of type III disease are often striking (see Figure 1). Palmar xanthomata are characterized by yellow/orange streaking of the palmar creases with soft tissue xanthomata either side of the skin crease. Tuberous xanthomata resemble cauliflower florets and develop on the elbows and knees. Sometimes tuberous xanthomata are surrounded by eruptive xanthomata.

Premature and extensive atherosclerosis is common and of interest is the occurrence of peripheral as well as coronary disease. In one series 30% had coronary artery disease and a similar proportion had peripheral vascular disease. If the triglycerides are particularly high then pancreatitis can occur.

Treatment. Contributing factors need to be identified and treated appropriately. Treatment is with diet and lifestyle measures together with hypolipidemic agents. Of interest in this patient, clofibrate (the first of the fibrate class of drugs) was used for about 9 years. The patient developed a now well known side effect of the compound, namely gallstones, because of cholesterol enrichment of the bile. However, type III disease does often respond well to fibrates and it is likely that this period of treatment was beneficial in retarding atherogenesis. Clofibrate is now redundant and cholelithiasis is not a problem with newer agents of the class.

Statins are also effective and they are the first choice treatment in the author's practice. Often combination therapy is necessary and statins may be combined with fibrates with relative safety. However, gemfibrozil should be avoided in combination with statins as this compound increases the plasma concentration of all statins. So, paradoxically, the fibrate with the most clinical trial outcome data is best avoided in combination with statins. With combination therapy this patient's lipid profile is largely satisfactory with normal cholesterol and LDL-cholesterol. His triglycerides remain slightly elevated and in this situation a useful secondary

107

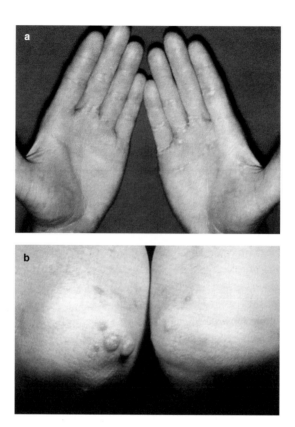

Figure 1 *(a) Palmar xanthomata typical of type III disease. (b) Tubero eruptive xanthomata on the elbows of a patient with type III disease.*

goal of therapy is nonHDL-cholesterol, which is satisfactory at 2.3 mmol/l. As his response to combination therapy has been so good, monotherapy with a higher dose of statin has not been tried.

The patient is monitored at intervals and at each visit he is questioned about possible drug side effects and cardiovascular symptoms, together with assessment of liver function and creatine phosphokinase. He is warned to stop the drugs in the event of severe muscle pain and tenderness which may indicate myositis.

Further reading

Mahley RW, Rall SC Jr. Type III hyperlipoproteinemia (dysbetalipoproteinemia; remnant particle disease). In: Betteridge, DJ, Illingworth, DR, Shepherd, J eds. Lipoproteins in Health and Disease. London: Arnold, 1999: 719–36.

Case 22

A Case For Measuring Apoprotein B

Beth Psaila and D John Betteridge

Case history

A 29-year-old man was referred to the Lipid Clinic by his primary care physician because of the finding of an abnormal lipid profile and a family history of dyslipidemia. He had no symptoms suggestive of cardiovascular disease. His only past medical history was of an episode of depression, treated for a short period with venlafaxine.

Interestingly, his sister had also been found to have dyslipidemia – with modestly raised triglycerides (2.4 mmol/l) and very low HDL-cholesterol (0.3 mmol/l). Both his mother (aged 57 years) and his mother's identical twin sister are being treated for hypertension, and his father (57 years) is alive. There is no known family history of premature atherosclerotic vascular disease, and no family history of diabetes.

He had never smoked, did not drink excess alcohol, and took regular exercise, enjoying mountain cycling and running. He ate a low-fat diet that was high in fruit and vegetables.

Examination was entirely normal with no stigmata of hyperlipidemia. Blood pressure was 130/79 and BMI 23.9 kg/m^2.

The fasting lipid profile was as follows: Total cholesterol, 4.5 mmol/l; triglycerides, 1.1 mmol/l; LDL-cholesterol, 3.3 mmol/l; HDL-cholesterol, 0.7 mmol/l; total-cholesterol/HDL-cholesterol ratio, 6.4. Apoprotein B was at the high end of the range at 1.25 g/l. Apoprotein A1 was low at 0.9 g/l. Renal, liver, and thyroid function were normal. Random glucose was 5.3. Protein electrophoresis and fibrinogen were normal. A diagnosis of probable familial combined hyperlipidemia (FCLH) was made. It can be seen that the main abnormality was a low HDL-cholesterol and this was reflected in a low apolipoprotein A1, a major alipoprotein of HDL. Alipoprotein B, the major alipoprotein of HDL, was higher than expected for the LDL-cholesterol concentration.

Familial combined hyperlipidemia

FCHL was first described in 1973 by Goldstein and colleagues in a study of myocardial infarction (MI) survivors and their families. This familial hyperlipidemia differed from heterozygous familial hypercholesterolemia (FH) in that affected individuals had raised cholesterol and raised triglyceride, raised cholesterol alone, or raised triglyceride alone in roughly equal numbers. Although originally thought to be an autosomal dominant condition, FCHL is now considered to show multigenic inheritance. There is as yet no useful genetic marker with which to identify the disease. Indeed, it is likely that FCHL will turn out to be a genetically heterogeneous disorder with strong gene and environment (overweight, lack of physical activity) interactions. This together with lack of specific physical signs such as tendon xanthomata found in FH means that formal diagnosis is imprecise, requiring detailed lipid analysis together with family studies. More recently FCHL has been shown to be associated with hypertension, insulin resistance, impaired glucose tolerance, and central obesity. FCHL is the most common form of heritable lipid disorder, with an estimated prevalence of 1–2%, and is found in about 20% of survivors of premature MI.

In FCHL there is overproduction of triglyceride-rich lipoproteins in the liver and the resulting phenotype will depend on other factors determining hydrolysis and clearance of particles of the VLDL/IDL/LDL cascade. Indeed a well-documented feature of FCHL is the notable variability in lipid and lipoprotein patterns, often with a low HDL-cholesterol both between family members and even within the individual patient over time. Consequently, diagnosis is often difficult and much of the recent literature on FCHL has focused on increasing diagnostic precision, primarily by including the measurement of apolipoprotein B.

Apolipoprotein B and lipoprotein particle numbers

Apolipoprotein B is the major protein of the VLDL/IDL/LDL cascade. Apolipoproteins are of paramount importance in lipid metabolism, not only in serving to transport insoluble lipid in the aqueous plasma environment, but also acting as ligands for receptor-mediated clearance of lipoproteins and regulators of enzyme activity.

As each lipoprotein particle of the cascade contains one molecule of apolipoprotein B its measurement provides a marker of lipid particle number.

The amount of LDL-cholesterol contained in each LDL particle is highly variable. FCHL is associated with a preponderance of smaller, denser particles.

110

Small dense LDL particles are depleted in lipid by almost half compared to more buoyant less dense particles. This leads to alteration of the accessibility of apolipoprotein B on the surface of the particle. This decreases the efficiency of binding to the LDL receptor and therefore clearance of the particle. In addition, these particles bind more avidly to glycosaminoglycans in the arterial wall. Small dense LDL are also more susceptible to oxidation. All of these factors may contribute to the increased atherogenicity attributed to this particle.

Regardless of cholesterol content, each LDL-cholesterol particle has one molecule of apolipoprotein B, therefore a raised apolipoprotein B out of proportion to the calculated LDL-cholesterol points to the presence of small, dense LDL. Accordingly, when small dense particles are present LDL-cholesterol does not provide a true reflection of the number of LDL particles.

Stalenhoef, Veerkamp and colleagues (Veerkamp et al 2002) have provided useful documentation of the variability in lipid phenotype in FCHL. At initial analysis, 31% of 299 subjects from 32 FCHL families were considered to be affected on the basis of total cholesterol and/or total triglyceride concentrations greater than the 90th percentile for the population. Five years later, when the same subjects were re-analysed using the same criteria, 26% of those originally thought to be affected based on cholesterol and triglyceride levels showed a normal lipid profile (i.e. total cholesterol and/or triglyceride < 90th percentile). On the other hand, 14% of those originally judged normal were subsequently re-classified as having FCHL. Thus a diagnosis of FCHL based on plasma total cholesterol and/or triglyceride levels is consistent in only 74% of subjects over a 5-year period and has low discriminatory power. Apolipoprotein B concentrations showed less variability over time and were more consistently associated with FCHL; affected subjects having a high apoprotein B even when total cholesterol and triglyceride levels were below the 90th percentile cut-off point.

Summary

FCHL is a highly significant and eminently treatable risk factor for premature atherosclerotic disease. It is characterized by an increase in total cholesterol and/or triglyceride levels, and a low HDL-cholesterol. However, these changes are highly variable both between family members and within an affected individual over time, posing a diagnostic conundrum. In addition, the LDL particles present may be cholesterol-depleted and thus measured LDL-cholesterol may be normal and may not reflect the increased number of atherogenic particles. The evidence suggests that diagnostic precision for diagnosing FCHL can be greatly increased if the measurement of apoprotein B is included in the assessment.

The standardization of apolipoprotein analysis within and between laboratories has improved enormously in recent years and there is no doubt that in the future increasing use will be made of these measurements, not only in diagnosis as in this case, but also in measuring response to treatment and in predicting CVD risk. It is clear from INTERHEART and other studies that the apolipoprotein B/apolipoprotein A1 ratio is probably the best predictor of vascular risk, accounting for approximately 50% of the vascular risk in a study across 52 countries involving approximately 30 000 subjects.

Further reading

Goldstein JL, Hazzard WR, Shrott HG et al. Hyperlipidaemia in coronary heart disease II. Genetic analysis of lipid levels in 176 families and delineation of new inherted disorder: combined hyperlipidemia. J Clin Invest 1973; 53: 1544–68.

Jarvik GP, Austin MA, Brunzell JD. Familial combined hyperlipidaemia. In: Betteridge DJ, Illingworth DR, Shepherd J, eds. Lipoproteins in Health and Disease. London: Arnold, 1999: 693–700.

Sniderman AD, Furberg CD, Keech A, Roeters van Lennep JE. Apoproteins versus lipids as indices of coronary risk and as targets for statin treatment. Lancet 2003; 361: 777–80.

Sniderman AD, Zhang XJ, Cianflone K. Governance of the concentration of plasma LDL: a reevaluation of the LDL receptor paradigm. Atherosclerosis 2000; 148: 215–29.

Veerkamp MJ, de Graaf J, Bredie SJH et al. Diagnosis of familial combined hyperlipidaemia based on lipid phenotype expression in 32 families. Arterioscler Thromb Vasc Biol 2002; 22: 274–82.

Yusuf S, Hawken S, Ounpuu S et al. for the INTERHEART Study investigators. Effect of potentially modifiable risk factors associated with myocardial infarction in 52 countries (the INTERHEART study): case control study. Lancet 2004; 364: 937–52.

Case 23

A HYPERCHOLESTEROLEMIC PATIENT WITH HYPOTHYROIDISM AND SOMETHING ELSE

Rafael Carmena and José T Real

Case report

A 42-year-old woman consulted her primary care physician because of the recent finding of a plasma total cholesterol value of 320 mg/dl and triglycerides of 63 mg/dl. She was asymptomatic and presented no symptoms of hypothyroidism; her menstrual cycles were regular. She was normotensive, had never smoked, did not drink alcohol, and was not diabetic.

She took no medications (nor contraceptives) and followed a typical Mediterranean diet: ingestion of about 2000 kcal/day with low cholesterol and saturated fat intake, and a correct amount (25% of daily energy) of polyunsaturated and mono-unsaturated fat.

She was an only child and both parents had died; the mother at age 85 of breast cancer and the father at age 45 of sudden death. The patient had no children (Figure 1).

On physical exam her body weight was 64 kg, height 168 cm, BMI 22.7, and waist circumference 72 cm. Blood pressure was 110/80 mm Hg and pulse was 74 regular. There was no goiter, no edema, and no jaundice. Tendon xanthomas and arcus were absent.

Once this initial exam was completed, the primary care physician decided to repeat some blood tests and evaluate new biological data. The results of these tests were as follows. Normal hemogram. Fasting plasma glucose 86 mg/dl, uric acid 4.2 mg/dl, creatinine 0.6 mg/dl, urea 45 mg/dl, AST 18, ALT 22, and total bilirubin 0.6. Lipids and lipoproteins: total cholesterol 394 mg/dl, triglycerides 73 mg/dl, HDL-cholesterol 64 mg/dl, LDL-cholesterol 312 mg/dl, and apoB 163 mg/dl.

A diagnosis of primary hypercholesterolemia was tentatively established (polygenic vs familial hypercholesterolemia) and treatment with 40 mg/day of simvastatin was started.

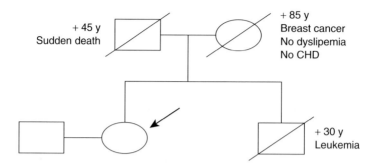

Figure 1 *Family tree of the patient.*

After 3 months, and with good compliance to diet and simvastatin treatment, the plasma lipids remained basically unchanged: total cholesterol 342 mg/dl, triglycerides 62 mg/dl, HDL-cholesterol 66 mg/dl, LDL-cholesterol 264 mg/dl, and apoB 153 mg/dl. The patient remained asymptomatic and did not complain of myalgia or loss of muscular strength.

At this point, the attending physician decided to exclude a secondary cause of hypercholesterolemia. Thyroid function tests were ordered and the results were: TSH, 19.2 mU/l; free-T4, 0.7 ng/dl. Anti-TPO antibodies were markedly elevated. A diagnosis of primary autoimmune hypothyroidism was made, simvastatin was discontinued, and treatment with escalating doses of levo-thyroxine was started. After 3 months of treatment and with a daily dose of 100 mcg of L-thyroxine for the preceding 2 months, a new blood test was obtained. The plasma lipid profile had changed very little: total cholesterol 282 mg/dl, triglycerides 56 mg/dl, HDL-cholesterol 63 mg/dl, LDL-cholesterol 206 mg/dl, and apoB 143 mg/dl.

The compliance to thyroid treatment was correct and the levels of TSH were 1.2 mU/l (see Figure 2). The diet had remained unchanged and no new drugs had been added to the treatment.

The primary care physician, at this point, thought again that the patient could also have a primary cause of hypercholesterolemia. The patient was referred to our Lipid Clinic, at the University Hospital in Valencia, for genetic diagnosis. The results of the genetic diagnosis showed a point mutation in exon 4 that confirmed the diagnosis of familial hypercholesterolemia (FH).

Comments

The clinical association between hypercholesterolemia and hypothyroidism in humans has been known since the 1920s; however, a clear molecular explanation

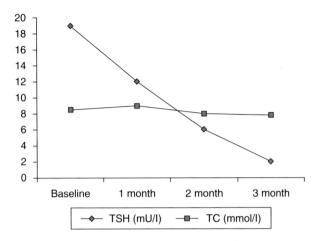

Figure 2 *Response to treatment with 100 mcg/day of levo-thyroxine. At 3 months, the TSH levels have normalized but the plasma total cholesterol (TC) values remain elevated.*

has been lacking for years.[1] Overt hypothyroidism is characterized by hypercholesterolemia and a marked increase in LDL and apolipoprotein B, because of a decreased fractional clearance of LDL by a reduced number of LDL receptors in the liver. The decrease in LDL receptor expression and increase in serum LDL-cholesterol associated with hypothyroidism could be explained by the effects of the thyroid hormone on SREBP-2.[2] SREBP-2 is known to regulate LDL receptor expression.

Hypothyroidism is often accompanied by diastolic hypertension that, in conjunction with the dyslipidemia, may promote atherosclerosis.[3]

Thyroxine therapy usually leads to a considerable improvement of the lipid profile. The changes in lipoproteins are correlated with changes in free thyroxine levels. When the adequate replacement therapy does not decrease the LDL-cholesterol plasma values other causes of hypercholesterolemia should be sought.[3] In the case of LDL-cholesterol values above the 95th percentile of our population, with normal renal and hepatic function, no intake of drugs capable of inducing hypercholesterolemia, and moderate–low saturated fat intake, it is important to consider primary causes of hypercholesterolemia. This was the fact in the patient reported, who presented autoimmune hypothyroidism and FH.

FH is rarely associated with autoimmune hypothyroidism. Hypothyroidism aggravates the FH phenotype, increasing coronary risk and exacerbating lipoprotein IIa phenotype. Hypothyroidism should be considered in FH subjects if LDL-cholesterol plasma values do not decrease as expected with diet therapy and the use of statins.[3] This was the case in our patient.

115

The use of statin treatment for hypercholesterolemia in an undiagnosed hypothyroid patient could increase the secondary effects of the statin, particularly myalgia and rhabdomyolysis.[3]

Finally, subclinical hypothyroidism does not appear to be associated with abnormalities in serum cholesterol or triglyceride levels when adjusted for confounding variables in a population-based study using NAHNES III population.[4]

References

1. Duntas LH. Thyroid disease and lipids. Thyroid 2002; 12: 287–93.
2. Shin DJ, Osborne TF. Thyroid hormone regulation and cholesterol metabolism are connected through Sterol Regulatory Element-Binding Protein-2 (SREBP-2). J Biol Chem. 2003; 278: 34114–18.
3. Roberts CG, Ladenson PW. Hypothyroidism. Lancet 2004; 363: 793–803.
4. Hueston WJ, Pearson WS. Subclinical hypothyroidism and the risk of hyper-cholesterolemia. Ann Fam Med 2004; 4: 351–5.

Case 24

DRY SKIN AND CARDIOVASCULAR HEALTH

Ioanna Gouni-Berthold and Wilhelm Krone

History

A 48-year-old engineer presented to his family physician for a routine check-up examination at the insistence of his wife who was worried about his heavy smoking (about one pack of cigarettes per day for the past 10 years). He was drinking four or five beers per week and was taking no medications. He had no physical complaints, except for some dryness of his skin. The physical exam was unremarkable except for an elevated blood pressure (BP) of 160/105 mm Hg. His body mass index (BMI) was 24.5 kg/m². He had no significant family history of cardiovascular disease (CVD). The laboratory values revealed a total cholesterol of 280 mg/dl, LDL-cholesterol 208 mg/dl, HDL-cholesterol 40 mg/dl, and Lp(a) 40 mg/dl. Otherwise the routine laboratory values, including (creatine kinase) CK, were unremarkable. An appointment with a dietician was scheduled for the coming week. During that visit his BP was found again to be elevated, so he was started on a diuretic and simvastatin 40 mg/day. Three weeks later he presented at his doctor's office complaining of severe, diffuse, muscle aches. In a blood test that was performed the same day the CK values were found to be increased (780 U/l, normal < 174 U/l). The LDL-cholesterol level was down to 170 mg/dl. His physician diagnosed a statin-induced myopathy, discontinued his statin immediately, and referred the patient to our outpatient clinic for further management.

The patient came to us 2 days after the withdrawal of simvastatin, quite worried and in a bad mood, since his muscle pains persisted. We routinely examine thyroid function tests in all patients presenting with hypercholesterolemia and/or elevated CKs. His serum TSH was 22 mU/l (normal values 0.27–4.2 mU/l), free T3 (FT3) 2.8 ng/l (normal values 1.8–4.6 ng/l), free T4 (FT4) 11.2 ng/l (normal values 9–15 ng/l). These values were confirmed in a repeat measurement two weeks later. Thyroid peroxidase antibodies (TPO) were positive at low titers (TPO 190 U/ml, normal < 100 U/ml). Based on the above evidence the diagnosis of subclinical hypothyroidism on the basis of autoimmune thyroiditis was established. After a

Table 1 Laboratory values before and after initiation of treatment with 100 µg/day LT4

Parameter	Before treatment with LT4	After 3 months treatment with LT4 (100 µg/day)
	Laboratory values	
TSH mU/l	22	3.6
FT3 (ng/l)	2.8	3.2
FT4 (ng/l)	10.8	12.3
Triglycerides (mg/dl)	160	182
Total cholesterol (mg/dl)	280	250
LDL-cholesterol (mg/dl)	208	174
HDL-cholesterol (mg/dl)	40	42
Lp(a) (mg/dl)	40	38
CK (U/l)	780	170

3 month treatment with L-thyroxine (LT4) 100 µg/day, his hypercholesterolemia improved, and the TSH levels normalized. His CK levels were normal and his muscle aches disappeared (see Table 1). He adamantly refused to be treated with a statin again, because of fear of recurrent myopathic symptoms, so treatment with the cholesterol absorption inhibitor ezetimibe 10 mg daily was initiated.

Discussion

Subclinical hypothyroidism (SH) is defined as a serum TSH concentration above the upper limit of the reference range with normal serum FT4 and FT3 concentrations. Most patients with SH (~70%) have no or few signs or symptoms of thyroid dysfunction. The overall prevalence of SH is about 4–10%, is higher in women, and increases with age. It reaches a peak of 21% in women and 16% in men over 74 years of age. Of patients with SH, approximately 2–5% progress to overt hypothyrodism. The rate of progression is proportional to the baseline serum TSH concentration and is higher in individuals with antithyroid antibodies (4.3% per year vs 2.6% per year in antibody-negative individuals). SH has been found in many studies to be associated with cardiac dysfunction, adverse cardiac endpoints (including atherosclerotic disease and cardiovascular mortality), elevations in total cholesterol and in LDL-cholesterol, and systemic hypothyroid and neuropsychiatric symptoms. Regarding the association between SH and hypertension, the evidence is sparse. Luboshitzky et al.[1] observed that mean diastolic BP was higher in 57 women with SH compared with 34 euthyroid controls (82 vs 75 mm Hg, $p < 0.01$). A potential mechanism for the diastolic hypertension of SH, which is reversible after treatment, is an increased peripheral vascular resistance. Furthermore, in patients with SH the flow-mediated endothelium-dependent vasodilation, a marker of endothelial dysfunction, has been shown to be impaired, as a result of decreased nitric oxide availability. This endothelial dysfunction is partially independent from dyslipidemia and can be reversed by LT4 supplementation. Two studies in the mid 1990s showed an increase in Lp(a) in SH. However, all other clinical trials, including two recent randomized placebo-controlled studies, found no significant differences in the Lp(a) concentrations between euthyroid subjects and patients with SH and no effect of LT4 treatment on its levels. Interestingly, unlike overt hypothyroidism, it has been clearly demonstrated by three case-control studies that there is no difference in homocysteine levels between SH and euthyroid controls, and no change in its levels after treatment. Regarding C-reative protein (CRP) levels in SH, Christ-Crain et al.[2] measured CRP levels in 63 patients with SH, compared them with 40 euthyroid controls and found them to be significantly higher in the SH group. However, the levels did not decrease after LT4 treatment and subsequent studies failed to reproduce these results.

The most compelling evidence linking SH to a greater cardiovascular risk came from the Rotterdam Study, published in 2000,[3] a cross-sectional analysis of 1149 women aged 55 years or older. Women with SH had a higher prevalence of aortic atherosclerosis on chest radiographs and a higher prevalence of myocardial infarction (MI) than euthyroid women after adjustment for age, BMI, HDL-cholesterol, BP, and smoking status. However, data from 3678 men and women enrolled in the Cardiovascular Health Study showed no differences between individuals with SH and euthyroid individuals in their prevalences of angina, MI, transient ischemic attack, stroke or peripheral arterial disease.

The hypercholesterolemia of untreated SH is most likely caused by reduced hepatic LDL particle clearance and has been shown to be reversible after treatment.[4] In general, the pathophysiology of hypercholesterolemia in SH and overt hypothyroidism is assumed to be the same. In hypothyroidism LDL-cholesterol has a prolonged half-life because of decreased catabolism, due to a decrease in the LDL receptor number. This effect is reversible with LT4 treatment. Molecular mapping has revealed functional thyroid response elements in the promoter region of the LDL receptor. A meta-analysis of 13 studies including data from 247 patients regarding the effects of LT4 therapy on cholesterol levels in SH published in 2000[5] showed that LT4 therapy decreases total cholesterol by a mean of 7.9 mg/dl and LDL-cholesterol by 10 mg/dl. Serum HDL-cholesterol and triglyceride concentrations showed no change. Later studies, such as a prospective, double-blind, placebo-controlled trial of 66 women with SH by Meier et al.,[6] demonstrated that LT4 replacement

119

significantly decreases total cholesterol and LDL-cholesterol concentrations (by 3.8% and 8.2%, respectively) after 12 months of treatment. Apolipoprotein B-100 (ApoB-100) concentrations were also significantly reduced. Triglycerides, HDL-cholesterol, and Lp(a) levels remained unchanged.

However, the levels did not decrease with LT4 treatment. Furthermore, in a recent study Monzani et al.[7] treated 45 patients (aged 37 ± 11 years) with SH with LT4 for 6 months. In comparison to 32 age- and sex-matched controls, patients with SH had elevated LDL-cholesterol and ApoB levels and higher mean intima-media thickness (IMT) values. In stepwise regression analysis, mean IMT was positively related to age, TSH, and LDL-cholesterol. LTsss replacement significantly reduced both total cholesterol and LDL-cholesterol (by 10% and 13%, respectively). The mean IMT was also significantly decreased by 11%. It seems therefore, that early carotid artery wall alterations are present in patients with SH and that LT4 treatment improves the lipid profile and the IMT thickness. While treatment of SH with LT4 has also been associated with improvement of symptoms, if present, there are no studies demonstrating that it decreases morbidity or mortality. The potential risks of therapy are limited to the development of subclinical hyperthyroidism, which may occur in 14–20% of individuals treated.

Of all the patients with SH, whom should we treat? The answer to this question is still under intense debate. A consensus statement of a panel of 13 experts published in *JAMA* in January 2004,[8] recommended treatment of SH only when the TSH levels are higher than 10 mU/l because of the associated elevations in serum cholesterol.

Interestingly, a consensus joint statement of the American Association of Clinical Endocrinologists, the American Thyroid Association, and the Endocrine Society published in the *Journal of Clinical Endocrinology and Metabolism* in 2005,[9] while agreeing with the aforementioned recommendations, goes even further and suggests that patients with mildly elevated TSH, namely between 4.5 and 10 mU/l, should also be considered for treatment, a recommendation which they base on the available data and the collective clinical experience of the panel.

Commentary

This case shows that before treating hypercholesterolemia with lipid-lowering medications, often associated with adverse side effects and significant costs, the physician should always exclude the presence of other underlying diseases that can either cause or exacerbate dyslipidemia, even when a relevant symptomatology is minimal or absent.

References

1. Luboshitzky R, Aviv A, Herer P, Lavie L. Risk factors for cardiovascular disease in women with subclinical hypothyroidism. Thyroid 2002; 12: 421–5.

2. Christ-Crain M, Meier C, Guglielmetti M. Elevated C-reactive protein and homocysteine values: cardiovascular risk factors in hypothyroidism? A cross-sectional and a double-blind, placebo-controlled trial. Atherosclerosis 2003; 166: 379–86.

3. Hak AE, Pols HA, Visser TJ. Subclinical hypothyroidism is an independent risk factor for atherosclerosis and myocardial infarction in elderly women: the Rotterdam Study. Ann Intern Med 2000: 15; 132: 270–8.

4. Caraccio N, Ferrannini MF. Lipoprotein profile in subclinical hypothyroidism: response to levothyroxine replacement, a randomized placebo-controlled study. J Clin Endocrinol Metab 2002; 87: 1533–8.

5. Danese MD, Ladenson PW, Meinert CL, Powe NR. Clinical review 115: effect of thyroxine therapy on serum lipoproteins in patients with mild thyroid failure: a quantitative review of the literature. J Clin Endocrinol Metab 2000; 85: 2993–3001. Review.

6. Meier C, Staub JJ, Roth CB et al. TSH-controlled l-thyroxine therapy reduces cholesterol levels and clinical symptoms in subclinical hypothyroidism: a double blind, placebo-controlled trial (Basel thyroid study). J Clin Endocrinol Metab 2001; 86: 4860–6.

7. Monzani F, Caraccio N, Kozakowa M et al. Effect of levothyroxine replacement on lipid profile and intima-media thickness in subclinical hypothyroidism: a double-blind, placebo-controlled study. J Clin Endocrinol Metab 2004; 89: 2099–106.

8. Col NF, Surks MI, Daniels GH. Subclinical thyroid disease: clinical applications. JAMA 2004; 291: 239–43.

9. Gharib H, Tuttle RM, Baskin HJ, et al. Subclinical thyroid dysfunction: a joint statement on management from the American Association of Clinical Endocrinologists, the American Thyroid Association, and the Endocrine Society. J Clin Endocrinol Metab 2005; 90: 581–5; discussion 586–7.

Case 25

ETHANOL-INDUCED COMBINED HYPERLIPIDEMIA

Juhani Kahri and Marja Riitta-Taskinen

Introduction

Hypertriglyceridemia is a risk factor for pancreatitis, and according to some authorities, also for coronary heart disease and other atherosclerotic complications.[1-3] Hypertriglyceridemia can be treated by weight loss through increased physical exercise and reduction of energy intake and dietary fat.[1,3] Hypolipidemic medication can also be considered, if high triglyceride values do not respond to lifestyle changes.

Ethanol consumption is a well recognized and common reason for secondary hypertriglyceridemia.[2] Therefore in clinical recommendations, patients with hypertriglyceridemia are generally advised to avoid alcohol, even if moderate alcohol consumption has proved to be cardioprotective.[3] We describe here a case of a middle-aged man, whose lipid values changed dramatically after he altered his beer-drinking habits.

Case history

The patient is a 42-year-old man who was otherwise healthy except for occasional allergic rhinitis in springtime. He was a former taxi driver but now he was unemployed. He stopped smoking 10 years ago. He went to a general practitioner for a routine health check. His serum cholesterol was 17.4 mmol/l (reference range < 5.0 mmol/l), triglyceride value was 64.7 mmol/l (reference range 0.45–2.6 mmol/l), aspartate aminotransferase (ASAT) was 171 U/l (reference range 15–45 U/l), alanine aminotransferase (ALAT) was 209 (reference range 10–50 U/l), and gammaglutamyltransferase (GGT) was 714 U/l (reference range 15–115 U/l). He was referred to the Cardiovascular Prevention Outpatient Clinic in the Helsinki University Central Hospital.

123

Table 1 Patient's lipoprotein and liver enzyme values before and after alcohol withdrawal

Parameter	Baseline	After 22 days
Cholesterol	19.4 mmol/l	5.2 mmol/l
Triglycerides	69.00 mmol/l	1.42 mmol/l
HDL-cholesterol	3.09 mmol/l	1.45 mmol/l
ASAT	139 U/l	62 U/l
ALAT	175 U/l	89 U/l
GT	901 U/l	367 U/l

At the examination his heart and lung auscultations were normal. Abdominal palpation was normal. No signs of tendon xanthomas or eruptive xanthomas were seen. The patient's height was 180 cm and weight was 87 kg (BMI 26.9 kg/m^2). The concentrations of serum total cholesterol and triglyceride were 19.4 mmol/l and 69.0 mmol/l, respectively. His HDL-cholesterol was clearly elevated, being 3.09 mmol/l. Serum transaminases are shown in Table 1. Bilirubin and conjugated bilirubin were normal. Serum creatinine and tyreotropin values were normal. Serology for hepatitis A, B, and C was negative. Serum antinuclear antibodies were normal. Abdominal ultrasound revealed no signs of extrahepatic biliary obstruction, but some signs of fatty liver were seen. When the patient was asked about his alcohol consumption, he admitted daily drinking of four to five pints (0.5 l) of beer containing 4.5% v/v of alcohol. Therefore he was advised not to consume alcoholic beverages in any form including beer. A revisit was scheduled in approximately 3 weeks. After 22 days of beer withdrawal, the patient's lipid values reached nearly normal levels (Table 1). LDL was 3.11 mmol/l. Based on the favorable results of the beer-poor diet, the patient was recommended to continue with the same diet and no hypolipidemic medication was started. However, the patient did not come to further appointments and therefore no information is available on his present status or history. Likewise studies to reveal potential causes of his severe dyslipidemia remain undone.

Discussion

Hypertriglyceridemia in an alcoholic patient is always an ambiguous issue. Ethanol-induced triglyceride elevations have been reported to be quite moderate in patients with hypertriglyceridemia.[1] Moderate drinking has been associated with beneficial effects on plasma lipoproteins: very low density lipoprotein

(VLDL) subfraction decreases and HDL subfraction increases.[4] Despite these favorable effects on the concentration of plasma HDL, and on the risk of coronary artery disease (CAD), alcohol is not normally advised to be used 'as a hypolipidemic drug' because of its otherwise detrimental effects on human health. Alcohol also increases serum triglyceride values and may cause secondary hyperlipidemia.[2,4] In particular, binge drinking does not always modify plasma lipoproteins in a favorable direction, and can actually increase triglyceride values.[5] Binge drinking also appears to negate the cardioprotective effects of moderate drinking.[5,6]

There are few studies of the effects of heavy consumption of alcohol on serum triglyceride values in hyperlipidemic patients. Our patient consumed at least 72–90 g of pure alcohol per day in the form of beer. Of note is that alcohol under-reporting is common and therefore actual intake remains inaccurate. On admission, he had very high serum triglyceride and cholesterol values as well as HDL-cholesterol, which normalized when the patient withdrew beer from his diet for 3 weeks.

There are several potential mechanisms behind the dramatic lipoprotein changes in our patient. His HDL-cholesterol was markedly elevated, as frequently seen in heavy drinkers without liver disease.[4] This finding is due to suspected alcohol-induced hypertriglyceridemia. Ethanol stimulates liver VLDL synthesis, which in clinical practice is seen as increases of serum triglyceride and also cholesterol concentrations. Acute ethanol ingestion has been reported to inhibit lipoprotein lipase (LPL) enzyme.[4] Therefore, it is possible in the present case that ethanol decreased the activity of LPL, and together with the overproduction of VLDL particles, the lipolytic capacity of plasma was exceeded causing chylomicronemic syndrome. The patient may also have a genetic deficiency of LPL or apoCII resulting in defective lipolysis. Carriers of LPL gene variants are prone to develop hypertriglyceridemia if VLDL production is exacerbated by other causes like heavy alcohol intake. Likewise familial combined hyperlipidemia (FCHL) may be a pre-existing abnormality associated with severe hypertriglyceridemia in connection with heavy alcohol intake. Since apoE phenotype was not determined for our patient, we cannot exclude the possibility that the patient exhibited apoE2/E2 phenotype, which is characterized by decreased binding of apoE to its remnant receptor,[7] leading to the accumulation of VLDL and chylomicron remnants in plasma, particularly in conditions where VLDL production is increased.

Alcohol use or abuse should be suspected behind marked hypertriglyceridemia, especially when it is combined with high cholesterol values. The impact of alcohol-induced rise of serum triglycerides on CAD risk is not clear. However, when serum triglyceride values exceed 10 mmol/l, the risk of acute pancreatitis becomes evident. Therefore it is warranted to advise patients with high triglyceride concentrations to avoid or to restrict ethanol in their diet.

References

1. Pownall HJ, Ballantyne CM, Kimball KT et al. Effect of moderate alcohol consumption on hypertriglyceridemia: a study in the fasting state. Arch Intern Med 1999; 159: 981–7.
2. Yadav D, Ptichumoni CS. Issues in hyperlipidemic pancreatitis. J Clin Gastroenterol 2003; 36: 54–62.
3. Expert Panel on Detection, Evaluation, and Treatment of High Blood Cholesterol in Adults. Executive Summary of the Third Report of the National Cholesterol Education Program (NCEP) Expert Panel on Detection, Evaluation, and Treatment of High Blood Cholesterol in Adults (Adult Treatment Panel III). JAMA 2001; 285: 2486–97.
4. Taskinen MR, Nikkilä EA, Välimäki M et al. Alcohol-induced changes in serum lipoproteins and in their metabolism. Am Heart J 1987; 113: 458–64.
5. Pletcher MJ, Varosy P, Kiefe CI et al. Alcohol consumption, binge drinking, and early coronary calcification: findings from the Coronary Artery Risk Development in Young Adults (CARDIA) Study. Am J Epidemiol 2005; 161: 423–33.
6. Li JM, Mukamal KJ. An update on alcohol and atherosclerosis. Curr Opin Lipidol 2004; 15: 673–80.
7. Mahley RW, Huang Y, Rall SC Jr. Pathogenesis of type III hyperlipoproteinemia (dysbetalipoproteinemia): questions, quandaries and paradoxes. J Lipid Res 1999; 40: 1933–49.

Case 26

A Patient With Type 2 Diabetes Mellitus

Kathryn CB Tan

Case study

The patient was an asymptomatic 60-year-old woman who was recently diagnosed as having type 2 diabetes mellitus. She was prompted to have a health check because her elder brother who was also a diabetic had just had a myocardial infarction at the age of 63. She was a nonsmoker and had a history of hypertension for 7 years and had been treated with a calcium channel blocker. There was a strong family history of type 2 diabetes. Her mother, elder brother, and a younger sister were diabetic. Physical examination showed that her weight and height were 69 kg and 157 cm, respectively. Blood pressure was 155/90 mm Hg. She had mild background retinopathy and the rest of the examination was unremarkable. Urinalysis showed 1 + glucose and 1 + proteinuria. Investigations showed a fasting glucose 10.5 mmol/l, HbA1c 9.2%, normal renal function, total cholesterol 6.0 mmol/l, fasting triglyceride 3.0 mmol/l, LDL-cholesterol 3.5 mmol/l, HDL-cholesterol 1.1 mmol/l, apolipoprotein (apo) AI 1.24 g/l, apoB 1.30 g/l, and proteinuria 0.5 g/day. ECG and exercise test were negative.

She was started on dietary therapy, metformin, and an angiotensin converting enzyme (ACE) inhibitor as well as aspirin. Six months later, she had lost 3 kg and her BP was 130/82 mm Hg. Her HbA1c had decreased to 7.2% and total cholesterol to 5.1 mmol/l, triglycerides 2.1 mmol/l, LDL-cholesterol 3.2 mmol/l, and HDL-cholesterol 1.0 mmol/l, apoAI 1.20 g/l, apoB 1.17 g/l. She was started on statin therapy and her lipid profile improved (total cholesterol 4.2 mmol/l, triglycerides 1.5 mmol/l, LDL-cholesterol 2.3 mmol/l, HDL-cholesterol 1.2 mmol/l).

She remained stable for over 2 years but she started to complain of lethargy and her weight increased. Her cholesterol had increased (total cholesterol 6.3 mmol/l, triglycerides 1.8 mmol/l, LDL-cholesterol 4.4 mmol/l, HDL-cholesterol 1.1 mmol/l) despite maintaining good diet and drug compliance.

The dosage of statin had remained the same over the 2-year period. Physical examination this time showed a small firm goiter. Her thyroid function test

127

showed low free T4 level, elevated TSH, and high titers of thyroid autoantibodies. She was commenced on thyroxine replacement for her hypothyroidism with improvement in her lipid profile.

Diabetic dyslipidemia

The lipid profile of this patient shows the typical abnormalities commonly seen in patients with type 2 diabetes mellitus. There are both quantitative and qualitative changes in plasma lipoproteins (Table 1) and dyslipidemia in type 2 diabetes is characterized by hypertriglyceridemia and a reduction in HDL, whereas LDL may be normal or elevated.[1] Hypertriglyceridemia is due to an increase in fasting and postprandial concentrations of triglyceride-rich lipoproteins and their atherogenic remnants. The increase in fasting triglyceride is due to an increase in VLDL, with abnormalities in both the production and clearance of VLDL. Postprandial lipemia is exaggerated and prolonged and is characterized by the long residence time of chylomicron and VLDL remnants in the circulation. Increased plasma triglyceride is almost invariably associated with reduced HDL levels in diabetes, as VLDL and HDL metabolism are closely linked. Not only is plasma concentration of HDL reduced (particularly HDL_2), the HDL particles are also dysfunctional and lead to inefficient reverse cholesterol transport. LDL-cholesterol may appear to be 'relatively normal' in diabetic patients but the distribution of LDL particles is altered with an increase in the proportion of the more atherogenic small dense LDL particles. As measurement of small dense LDL is not widely available, the LDL-cholesterol level in the context of plasma apoB level can be used to help to determine the presence or absence of small dense LDL particles, and an elevated plasma apoB level reflects increased number of LDL particles. Lipoprotein metabolism is influenced by glycemic control in type 2 diabetes and improvement in diabetic control, irrespective of the mode of treatment used, will usually result in some degree of improvement in plasma lipid levels.

Management of diabetic dyslipidemia

Lipid management is aimed at lowering LDL and triglyceride and raising HDL, and lipid-lowering agents are frequently required in addition to dietary intervention. Statins are currently the class of lipid-lowering agents that have shown the most convincing effect on cardiovascular protection.[2] Subgroup analysis of diabetic

128

Table 1 Quantitative changes in plasma lipids and apolipoproteins in type 2 diabetes

Parameter	Good control	Poor control
Plasma cholesterol	N/↑	↑
Plasma triglyceride	N/↑	↑↑
LDL-cholesterol	N/↑	↑
HDL-cholesterol	↓	↓
Apolipoprotein A	N/↓	↓
Apolipoprotein B	N/↑	↑

subjects from early statin trials suggested that lowering cholesterol reduced cardiovascular events. Since then, numerous other trials of statin treatment have been reported, with randomized data available on over 18 000 persons with diabetes. Results from the recent Heart Protection Study and the Collaborative Atorvastatin Diabetes Study have clearly confirmed that statin therapy significantly reduced the risk of major cardiovascular events in patients with diabetes in terms of both primary and secondary prevention. In contrast to statin therapy, less data are available on the magnitude of benefits of treating diabetic dyslipidemia with fibrates. The use of gemfibrozil in the Helsinki Heart Study and the Veterans Affairs High-density Lipoprotein Cholesterol Intervention Trial is associated with a reduction in cardiovascular endpoints. However, the recent Fenofibrate Intervention and Event Lowering in Diabetes (FIELD) Study failed to show overall treatment benefits with a fibrate. Hence, first-line therapy should remain statins and not fibrates in diabetic patients.

Based on the large body of evidence showing that statin therapy significantly reduces cardiovascular morbidity and mortality in patients with type 2 diabetes, there is now strong agreement across international guidelines on the recommendation of aggressive lipid-lowering therapy in diabetic patients, although there may be minor differences between guidelines on cholesterol goals. In the recent update of the National Cholesterol Education Program – Adult Treatment Panel III guidelines, an appropriate threshold for initiation of LDL-cholesterol-lowering therapy in individuals with diabetes is ≥ 2.6 mmol/l, with an option to lower LDL to a target of < 1.8 mmol/l for the very high-risk individual. In younger diabetic patients without additional risk factors who have a moderately high cardiovascular risk, the threshold for institution of LDL-lowering therapy is 3.4 mmol/l.

This patient's LDL was 3.2 mmol/l and apoB level remained elevated despite lifestyle modification and improvement in her glycemic control. She also had hypertension and proteinuria. Her absolute risk of coronary heart disease was high and statin therapy was warranted. This case also illustrates the multifactorial approach in the management of patients with diabetes. In addition to treating dyslipidemia, the aggressive pursuit of other risk factor goals in diabetic patients is equally important. The multiple risk factor approach includes nutrition therapy, weight reduction when indicated, increased physical activity, and improving glycemic control with oral agents or insulin, with careful monitoring and aggressive management of other risk factors like hypertension and albuminuria. Multifactorial intervention has been shown to reduce the risk of cardiovascular events in diabetic patients.[3]

This case also reminds us that hypothyroidism is an important cause of secondary dyslipidemia and is common in patients with diabetes and in the elderly population. In the presence of elevated LDL, thyroid function should be checked to rule out hypothyroidism because classical clinical features of hypothyroidism are often absent – especially in the elderly. Hypothyroidism is most commonly linked to hypercholesterolemia due to increased LDL concentrations but abnormalities in triglyceride and HDL levels can also occur. Thyroid hormone modulates LDL receptor activity, thus leading to changes in plasma LDL levels. The activities of lipolytic enzymes are also influenced by thyroid hormones and reduction in enzyme activities in hypothyroidism leads to increases in triglyceride levels. These changes are reversible upon treatment of the underlying thyroid disorder.

References

1. Taskinen MR. Diabetic dyslipidemia: from basic research to clinical practice. Diabetologia 2003; 46: 733–49.
2. Armitage J, Bowman L. Cardiovascular outcomes among participants with diabetes in the recent large statin trials. Curr Opin Lipidol 2004; 15: 439–46.
3. Gaede P, Vedel P, Larsen N et al. Multifactorial intervention and cardiovascular disease in patients with type 2 diabetes. N Engl J Med 2003; 348: 383–93.

A Modicum Of Suspicion: Diabetic Kidney Disease And Dyslipidemia

Merlin C Thomas and Per-Henrik Groop

Case history

A 58-year-old man is admitted to his local hospital with a progressive history of shortness of breath. He has felt this way for some weeks, but over the last few days he has become increasingly breathless. He denies any chest pain or palpitations. He claims to have been fit and well up until the last few months with 'just a touch of diabetes' as his only problem.

His first contact with the hospital had been 8 years previously, when he was referred for urological investigation. The referral letter described the patient complaining of nocturia and impotence. Rectal examination revealed an enlarged smooth prostate. His blood pressure at this clinic visit was noted to be elevated at 170/90 mm Hg. He admitted to being somewhat anxious in coming to the hospital.

He presented for elective transurethral surgery 6 months later. On the day of the operation he was reviewed by an anesthetist. On examination, he was noted to be a 'short round man' weighing 104 kg and measuring 165 cm in height. His supine blood pressure was 155/90 mm Hg. The remainder of his clinical examination was noted to be unremarkable. Preoperative blood tests showed an albumin 36 g/l, urea of 9.2 mmol/l, creatinine of 120 μmol/l (hospital laboratory normal range 50–120 μmol/l). A ward urinalysis on the morning of surgery was positive for protein and glucose.

Following the operation, he was referred back to his general practitioner (GP) for further investigations. His blood pressure was elevated at 180/90 mm Hg with no orthostatic change. The GP noted white cells and protein in his urine following his surgery. Random capillary testing showed elevated blood glucose at a level of 8.2 mmol/l. His cholesterol was 5.5 mmol/l with LDL-cholesterol of 3.5 and triglycerides of 2.6 mmo/l. His HDL-cholesterol was 0.8 mmol/l. At this time he was informed that he should lose weight, improve his diet, and exercise more often. He was also commenced on atenolol 50 mg a day for his blood pressure, based on guidelines that suggest starting with a beta-blocker or diuretic in patients with uncomplicated hypertension.

Following the prescribed diet and exercise regime, he lost 6 kg over the next year. His blood glucose measurements were between 6 and 9 mmol/l every time he saw his GP, although his HbA_{1c} remained elevated at 9%. At follow-up visits his systolic blood pressure remained around 145–155 mm Hg and the daily dose of atenolol was doubled. His total cholesterol fell with his lifestyle changes, although his triglycerides remained elevated at 2.3 mmol/l and his HDL-cholesterol remained low at 0.8 mmol/l. He then moved away, presenting again only prior to his hospital admission with shortness of breath.

Examination at the time of his admission reveals an obese man weighing 115 kg. His blood pressure is 165/85 and blood sugar 13.6 mmol/l. He is clinically in biventricular failure with pitting edema and bilateral lung crepitations with a left-sided pleural effusion. An electrocardiogram demonstrates atrial fibrillation with T wave inversion across the anterior leads with inferior Q waves without acute ST changes. An echocardiogram confirms his poor cardiac function with inferior akinesis and significant left ventricular hypertrophy. He has reduced sensation to pinprick and light touch over his lower limbs. He has a left femoral bruit and absent pedal pulses. Fundoscopy shows grade II hypertensive changes with a number of soft exudates.

His creatinine is now 250 µmol/l with a urea of 19 mmol/l. His potassium is 5.5 mmol/l. Urinalysis shows ++ proteinuria. His blood HbA_{1c} is 8.3%; his total cholesterol is elevated at 7.8 mmol/l; LDL-cholesterol, 153 mg/dl (4.0 mmol/l); HDL-cholesterol, 36 mg/dl (0.93 mmol/l); triglyceride level, 350 mg/dl (4.0 mmol/l); HDL/total cholesterol ratio 0.12. An angiogram is performed, which shows diffuse atherosclerotic disease of both the left anterior descending and right coronary arteries with multiple stenoses and an occluded dominant circumflex artery. He is placed on the waiting list for coronary bypass grafting. However, 4 months later he collapses and dies of an apparent massive myocardial infarction (MI).

Commentary

There seems little doubt that cases such as this one will become increasingly common in adult medicine. More than 11 million Americans have both diabetes and hypertension. Many of these already have or will develop renal and cardiovascular damage.[1] Dyslipidemia is also an important element of this multi-component metabolic disorder, both as a marker for disease/risk and a target for intervention.

A range of quantitative and qualitative lipid and lipoprotein abnormalities are observed in patients with diabetes. The main components of diabetic dyslipidemia are excessive postprandial lipemia associated with increased plasma triglycerides, small dense LDL, and reduced HDL-cholesterol levels.[2] Increased triglyceride levels are largely due to the accumulation of very low density lipoprotein (VLDL), chylomicron remnants, and intermediate density lipoprotein (IDL) particles in the plasma. This is thought to reflect both the overproduction of triglyceride-rich VLDL (due to increased flux of free fatty acids and hepatic resistance to the effects of insulin), together with reduced catabolism (associated with reduced lipoprotein lipase activity).[3] LDL-cholesterol levels in patients with type 2 diabetes are, as in this case, usually within the normal range. However, there remain significant disturbances in LDL metabolism in diabetes. For example, LDL production is significantly reduced, while impaired turnover of LDL particles[4] promotes glycoxidative modification of lipoprotein particles and cholesterol deposition in the arterial wall. Diabetes is also associated with the accumulation of small dense, triglyceride-rich LDL particles,[3] that have an increased atherogenic potential.[5] HDL-cholesterol levels are invariably reduced in patients with type 2 diabetes, reflecting increased catabolism of HDL particles. In addition, HDL particles become enriched with triglycerides, in an attempt to cope with an increased VLDL burden. This may be partly responsible for their increased catabolism.[4]

The finding of dyslipidemia, particularly that associated with a high triglyceride level and reduced HDL-cholesterol (and in an obese male!), should always lead to a formal test for diabetes. Either a fasting plasma glucose (FPG) test or 2-hour oral glucose tolerance test (OGTT, 75 g glucose load) is appropriate. The FPG test may be more convenient to patients, less costly, more reproducible, and easier to administer than the 2-hour OGTT.[6] The 2-hour OGTT is more sensitive and specific, and is also able to identify individuals with impaired glucose tolerance, who are at increased risk for the development of diabetes and cardiovascular disease. Stratification of cardiovascular risk is an important part of adult medicine, and a diagnosis of diabetes made appropriately some years before his first MI should have provided a call for action.

Although the finding of dyslipidemia in a patient with diabetes is commonplace, it should also prompt the consideration of possible secondary factors, particularly those that may be responsive to intervention. In many cases, dietary excesses and inactivity directly contribute to dyslipidemia and are amenable to lifestyle interventions.[7] In other individuals, uncontrolled blood sugar levels may directly contribute to hypertriglyceridemia, which may be partly corrected along with the restoration of glycemic control. The presence of dyslipidemia in a patient with diabetes should also prompt the consideration of diabetic renal disease, and *vice versa*. Dyslipidemia is even more severe in patients who have diabetes and nephropathy. The early stages of diabetic nephropathy are associated with further elevated triglyceride levels and reduced levels of HDL-cholesterol. With the development of overt nephropathy, these changes are compounded. Moreover, the amount of albuminuria is closely associated with the average LDL particle size in type 2 diabetes,[8] and may contribute to a variable elevation in the levels of LDL-cholesterol.[9] Ultimately, declining renal function sees further qualitative lipoprotein modifications, that are more severe than seen in nondiabetic patients with chronic kidney disease.

An accurate assessment of the severity of diabetic renal disease should have been an important component of the management of this individual. In hindsight, this patient had overt nephropathy with proteinuria detectable on dipstick and renal impairment. Certainly, it was easy to attribute the clinical findings in this case to other causes (recent surgery, hypertension, urosepsis, etc.) but one must always have a modicum of suspicion for underlying renal disease. Screening for diabetic nephropathy should be initiated at the time of diagnosis in patients with type 2 diabetes, since ~7% of them already have microalbuminuria. However, even in those individuals not known to have diabetes, those with dyslipidemia should undergo urine analysis and have an estimation of creatinine clearance/glomerular filtration rate (GFR).

An early diagnosis is the cornerstone upon which the prevention of diabetic complications rests. The first step in the screening and diagnosis of diabetic nephropathy is to measure albumin in a spot urine sample, collected either as the first urine in the morning or at random, for example, at the medical visit. Although this method is accurate and easy to perform, it requires a level of suspicion to make the correct diagnosis. In this case the physician believed that urinary protein loss was a result of asymptomatic urinary tract infection (UTI). However, asymptomatic UTI does not appear to increase albumin excretion rate (AER) in patients with type 2 diabetes.[10] Nonetheless, it is still recommended that the AER be determined after resolution of UTI to avoid falsely elevated results. Regardless, all abnormal tests should be confirmed in two out of three samples collected over a 3–6-month period, due to the known day-to-day variability in AER. It should also be noted that not all albuminuria in diabetes is due to diabetic nephropathy. Certainly, urinary retention may be associated with albuminuria, which can persist for some months after its resolution.[11] Smoking, uncontrolled hypertension, and heart failure are also associated with albuminuria.[12] Nonetheless, AER remains an important risk factor for cardiac risk, and an important target for intervention.

There are some patients with diabetes in whom renal function declines despite the absence of overt microvascular disease. For example, in NHANES III (Third National Health and Nutrition Examination Survey), moderate to severe renal impairment ($< 60 \, \text{ml/min}/1.73 \, \text{m}^{-2}$) was present in 30% of patients with type 2 diabetes ($n = 1197$) in the absence of micro- or macroalbuminuria and retinopathy.[13] There is no evidence that these patients do not have diabetic nephropathy. Moreover, their clinical behavior is similar to that seen in patients with albuminuria and a similar degree of renal impairment. Consequently, GFR should be routinely estimated and urinary albumin excretion (UAE) should be routinely measured for a proper screening of diabetic nephropathy. An isolated serum creatinine concentration should not be used as the sole indicator of renal function, particularly when evaluating creatinine measurements in the context of so-called 'normal concentration ranges'.[14] Substantial damage can occur with very little change in serum creatinine due to compensatory hyperfiltration in remaining nephrons. Clearance estimated from urinary creatinine collections may also prove inaccurate due to incomplete urine collection and overestimation of the GFR at low levels of renal function (due to increased tubular secretion of creatinine). This can only be partly corrected using an average of urea and creatinine clearance.[15] A calculated GFR (using formulae such as those employed in the Modification of Diet in Renal Disease (MDRD) Study[16] or the Cockroft-Gault), with correction for body surface area, allows a better estimation of renal function. However, such formulae may still be insensitive to early damage and inaccurate at extremes of body mass. In our case, both the Cockroft-Gault (55 ml/min) and the extended MDRD formula (53 ml/min), would have documented renal impairment at the time of first presentation. Along with the presence of proteinuria, this should have identified this patient as being at significant risk of cardiovascular disease.

Dyslipidemia is more than a marker of diabetic renal disease. There is strong evidence that it is also an important risk factor for diabetic nephropathy. For example, moderately elevated lipid levels, especially when combined with high-normal blood pressure and raised HbA_{1c} levels, have been associated with progression of diabetic nephropathy.[17] Although aggressive treatment of dyslipidemia in patients with diabetic nephropathy has beneficial effects on macrovascular disease, its impact on microvascular disease remains controversial and the impact of lipid reduction on progression of diabetic nephropathy is still unknown. There is some evidence that antilipemic agents might preserve GFR and decrease proteinuria in diabetic individuals. For example, in the Heart Protection Study, 40 mg simvastatin reduced the rate of GFR decline by 25% in patients with diabetes.[18] This effect was independent of cholesterol-lowering effects. In the GREek Atorvastatin and Coronary heart disease Evaluation (GREACE) study patients with diabetes allocated to atorvastatin therapy had a 10.9% increase in GFR.[19] A recent meta-analysis showed that lipid lowering was associated with a slower rate of the decline of renal function compared with control patients, which was comparable to the beneficial effect of an ACE inhibitor on preservation of renal function.[20] Although renal protection is not currently an indication for lipid-lowering therapy, dyslipidemia in patients with diabetic renal disease should be managed aggressively, according to current guidelines, to prevent macrovascular disease and potentially benefit microvascular complications.

135

It has also been suggested that lipid lowering may reduce the risk of developing type 2 diabetes mellitus, in patients with impaired glucose tolerance. For example, in the West of Scotland Coronary Prevention Study (WOSCOPS) treatment with pravastatin was associated with a 30% reduction in the hazard of developing diabetes.[21] Similarly, in a retrospective cohort study in patients with diabetes newly started on oral antidiabetic agents, the use of statins was associated with a delay in starting insulin treatment.[22] A number of mechanisms contribute to the development and progression of type 2 diabetes.[23] One pathway appears to be chronic exposure of the β-cell to elevated free fatty acid (FFA) concentrations (so-called lipotoxicity), which in the presence of elevated glucose levels, results in impaired insulin expression and secretion and increased β-cell apoptosis.[24–27] To this end control of dyslipidemia may also be an important component to delay the onset or slow the progression of diabetes itself.

The clinical management of any patient with diabetes should be mindful of the complex and often confounding interactions that exist between risk factors and adverse outcomes. For example, renal disease is considered a risk factor for retinopathy. This association is not causal as both may be considered manifestations of the same disease process. In so far as dyslipidemia may also be a manifestation of renal disease in diabetes, successful management of lipid levels in diabetes is also dependent on the control of renal disease, and in particular, proteinuria. Indeed, abnormalities in lipid and lipoprotein disturbances may be more closely related to albuminuria than to cardiovascular disease in patients with diabetes. Although it is generally thought that blockade of the renin angiotensin system (RAS) has neutral effects on the metabolic profile, interventions to slow the progression of renal disease (and reduce urinary protein excretion) are also able to significantly improve lipid profiles at all stages of diabetic nephropathy. For example, blockade of the RAS, achieved by ACE inhibition or angiotensin receptor blockade, reduces the atherogenic lipid profile in patients with type 2 diabetes and microalbuminuria, and correlates with reductions in UAE.[28,29] Similarly, in patients with proteinuria and/or renal impairment, blockade of the RAS has beneficial effects on serum levels of total cholesterol and lipoprotein (a).[30] Such renoprotective interventions may be the most efficient way to correct dyslipidemia in some patients with diabetic nephropathy, particularly those who do not meet (*cholesterol-centric*) criteria for intervention with statin therapy. Although a beta-blocker was used in this patient (because neither diabetes nor nephropathy were suspected), successful management of urinary protein loss at the time of diagnosis might have restored lipid levels to the normal range. Indeed, the lower the level of proteinuria that can be achieved by therapy the greater the eventual benefit in terms of long-term outcome.[31] To this end, albuminuria and not blood pressure should be considered the key target for intervention and medical treatments should be incremented accordingly to achieve the greatest levels of albuminuria reduction.

136

For the management of elevated triglyceride levels in diabetes, hyperglycemia must first be controlled before embarking on pharmacological therapies. Sometimes that can be achieved by lifestyle changes including regular physical activity, weight loss, smoking cessation, and dietary modification, and allows many patients to achieve target levels for metabolic control. In particular, weight reduction in patients with obesity reduces cardiovascular risk and improves metabolic control.[32] Increased physical activity decreases triglyceride levels and may increase HDL-cholesterol levels, over and above improvements in glycemic control.

Some patients will be unable to achieve or sustain near normoglycemia without oral antidiabetic agents or insulin. Both sulfonylureas and metformin are effective in reducing blood glucose in most patients. Metformin is often preferred for obese patients and those with elevated cholesterol or triglycerides. However, in the presence of renal impairment (even though the serum creatinine is in the normal range) caution should be exercised with metformin. In addition, in patients with reduced renal function, sulfonylureas with predominant hepatic clearance (e.g. tolbutamide) may be preferred over those with renal excretion (e.g. glibenclamide). Recent data suggest that thiazolidinedione drugs (PPARγ agonists), which improve both insulin sensitivity and lipid parameters, may be useful in this setting.[33] However, more evidence is needed regarding long-term safety for this class of agents to be accepted as first-line therapy for diabetic dyslipidemia.

For patients with dyslipidemia not meeting targets for lipid levels, additional pharmacological intervention may be appropriate. There are some data supporting the use of HMG-CoA reductase inhibitors, niacin or fibrates to achieve lipid targets.[34]

A number of studies have shown that fibrates confer a beneficial effect in patients with diabetes. In the Veterans Affairs High-Density Lipoprotein Intervention Trial (VA-HIT), the subgroup of patients with diabetes treated with gemfibrozil had reduced the risk of a composite endpoint of coronary heart disease (CHD) death, stroke or MI by 32% and reduced CHD deaths by 41% compared with those with diabetes receiving standard care.[35] The Diabetes Atherosclerosis Intervention Study (DAIS) showed that 3 years of treatment with fenofibrate resulted in significant reductions in angiographic progression of atherosclerosis and stenosis ($p \leq 0.03$).[36] However, in the Helsinki Heart Study, among patients with diabetes, although gemfibrozil reduced the incidence of primary CHD compared with placebo (3.4 vs 10.5%), this difference was not statistically significant.[37] Although effective in patients with diabetes, it must be noted that fibrates should be avoided in moderate or severe renal failure because of the risk of rhabdomyolysis.[38]

In general, niacin has not been considered useful in patients with type 2 diabetes because of its deleterious effects on insulin resistance in moderate–high

137

dose. However, niacin increases HDL levels more than do fibrates. In addition, niacin increases the anti-atherogenic lipoprotein, Lp(A-I). However, it remains to be established whether increasing HDL or Lp(A-1) in the presence of optimal LDL control is more beneficial than LDL-lowering therapy alone. Certainly, low-dose or extended-release niacin can be used effectively and safely in patients with type 2 diabetes mellitus, who often have low HDL levels. Niacin may also be useful in combination with statins, without the added risk of rhabdomyolysis associated with a fibrate–statin combination. Nonetheless, in patients with poor sugar control or those with renal impairment, niacin should be avoided.

There is strong evidence for the use of statins in patients with diabetes. In the Scandinavian Simvastatin Survival (4S) and the Cholesterol and Recurrent Events (CARE) studies, patients with type 2 diabetes achieved significant reductions in mortality and cardiovascular disease following statin therapy.[39,40] The MRC/BHF Heart Protection Study (HPS) demonstrated that statin treatment reduced the rate of first major vascular events by about a quarter in those with diabetes, although the risk associated with diabetes was not eliminated.[41] Current guidelines mandate lowering of LDL levels to < 2.6 mmol/l (100 mg/dl) as the primary goal of lipid-lowering therapy in patients with diabetes. Although other lipid parameters have atherogenic effects, there is strong evidence that LDL lowering in diabetes is associated with improved clinical outcomes.[42] Indeed, the Collaborative Atorvastatin Diabetes Study (CARDS), which showed a reduction of cardiovascular events in patients with diabetes, suggested that all diabetic patients should be taking statins.[43] Although there is a strong rationale for this kind of catch-all approach, each patient should be carefully assessed and treated according to their risk. In the case detailed above (an obese male, with overt nephropathy, hypertension, and renal impairment), attaining an LDL goal of < 70 mg/dl would be appropriate, and would almost certainly necessitate a statin agent. Moreover, the so-called 'pleiotropic effects' of statins 'beyond cholesterol lowering' may influence cell proliferation, thrombosis, inflammation, endothelial function, and immunomodulation, pathways that play a role in atherogenesis and microvascular damage. Certainly, when both LDL-cholesterol and triglycerides are elevated, as in this case, statins should be considered the best choice. The best approach to patients with isolated hypertriglyceridemia remains to be determined. Among statins, atorvastatin has been seen to be of particular utility in patients with diabetic renal disease, owing to its ability to reduce triglycerides and its predominant liver excretion.[44] However, in the presence of moderate or severe renal failure, particular attention should be paid to monitoring for statin-induced rhabdomyolysis.

In summary, silent renal disease in diabetes, like silent myocardial ischemia, is important to recognize and treat early. Many of the interventions recommended for the prevention of diabetic complications are more efficacious the earlier they are initiated, particularly before overt disease becomes established. The key trouble is

138

that type 2 diabetes is often present many years before a diagnosis of diabetes is finally made. Dyslipidemia is an important clue to underlying renal disease, as it is a potent risk factor for vascular complications in patients with diabetes. Early intervention is the cornerstone of the management of diabetic nephropathy. However, even late in the game, aggressive management of lipids in overt nephropathy may still prevent cardiovascular events and premature mortality.

References

1. Bakris GL, Williams M, Dworkin L et al. Preserving renal function in adults with hypertension and diabetes: a consensus approach. National Kidney Foundation Hypertension and Diabetes Executive Committees Working Group. Am J Kidney Dis 2000; 36(3): 646–61.

2. Verges B. Diabetic dyslipidaemia: insights for optimizing patient management. Curr Med Res Opin 2005; 21 (Suppl 1): S29–S40.

3. Taskinen MR. Diabetic dyslipidaemia: from basic research to clinical practice. Diabetologia 2003; 46: 733–49.

4. Duvillard L, Florentin E, Lizard G et al. Cell surface expression of LDL receptor is decreased in type 2 diabetic patients and is normalized by insulin therapy. Diabetes Care 2003; 26: 1540–4.

5. Chait A, Brazg RL, Tribble DL, Krauss RM. Susceptibility of small, dense, low-density lipoproteins to oxidative modification in subjects with the atherogenic lipoprotein phenotype, pattern B. Am J Med 1993; 94: 350–6.

6. Expert Committee on the Diagnosis and Classification of Diabetes Mellitus: Follow-up report on the diagnosis of diabetes mellitus. Diabetes Care 2003; 26: 3160–7.

7. American Diabetes Association. Evidence-based nutrition principles and recommendations for the treatment and prevention of diabetes and related complications (Position statement). Diabetes Care 2003; 26(Suppl 1): S51–S61.

8. Yoshino G, Hirano T, Kazumi T. Atherogenic lipoproteins and diabetes mellitus. J Diabetes Complications 2002; 16: 29–34.

9. Wheeler DC, Bernard DB. Lipid abnormalities in the nephrotic syndrome: causes, consequences, and treatment. Am J Kidney Dis 1994; 23: 331–46.

10. Hernandez C, Simo R. Albumin excretion rate is not affected by asymptomatic urinary tract infection: a prospective study. Diabetes Care 2004; 27(7): 1565–9.

11. Mustonen S, Ala-Houhala I, Tammela TL. Proteinuria and renal function during and after acute urinary retention. J Urol 1999; 161(6): 1781–4; discussion 1784–5.

12. Pinto-Sietsma SJ, Mulder J, Janssen WM et al. Smoking is related to albuminuria and abnormal renal function in nondiabetic persons. Ann Intern Med 2000; 133(8): 585–91.

139

13. Kramer HJ, Nguyen QD, Curhan G, Hsu CY. Renal insufficiency in the absence of albuminuria and retinopathy among adults with type 2 diabetes mellitus. JAMA 2003; 289: 3273–7.

14. Shah BV, Levey AS. Spontaneous changes in the rate of decline in reciprocal serum creatinine: errors in predicting the progression of renal disease from extrapolation of the slope. J Am Soc Nephrology 1992; 2: 1186–91.

15. Ruggeneti P. Chronic proteinuric nephropathies: outcomes and response to treatment in a prospective cohort of 352 patients with different patterns of renal injury. Am J Kidney Dis 2000; 35: 1155–65.

16. Peterson JC, Adler S, Burkart JM et al. Blood pressure control, proteinuria, and the progression of renal disease. The Modification of Diet in Renal Disease Study. Ann Intern Med 1995; 123: 754–62.

17. Groop PH, Elliott T, Ekstrand A et al. Multiple lipoprotein abnormalities in type I diabetic patients with renal disease. Diabetes. 1996; 45: 974–9.

18. Heart Protection Study Collaborative Group. MRC/BHF Heart Protection Study of cholesterol-lowering with simvastatin in 5963 people with diabetes: a randomised placebo-controlled trial. Lancet 2003; 361: 2005–16.

19. Athyros VG, Mikhailidis DP, Papageorgiou AA et al. The effect of statins versus untreated dyslipidemia on renal function in patients with coronary heart disease. A subgroup analysis of the Greek atorvastatin and coronary heart disease evaluation (GREACE) study. J Clin Pathol 2004; 57(7): 728–34.

20. Fried LF, Orchard TJ, Kasiske BL. Effect of lipid reduction on the progression of renal disease: a meta-analysis. Kidney Int 2001; 59(1): 260–9.

21. Freeman D, Norrie J, Sattar N et al. Pravastatin and the development of diabetes mellitus: evidence for a protective treatment effect in the West of Scotland Coronary Prevention Study. Circulation 2001; 103: 357–62.

22. Yee A, Majumdar SR, Simpson SH et al. Statin use in Type 2 diabetes mellitus is associated with a delay in starting insulin. Diabetic Med 2004; 21(9): 962–7.

23. Stumvoll M, Goldstein BJ, van Haeften TW. Type 2 diabetes: principles of pathogenesis and therapy. Lancet 2005; 365(9467): 1333–46.

24. Zhou YP, Grill V. Long term exposure to fatty acids and ketones inhibits B-cell functions in human pancreatic islets of Langerhans. J Clin Endocrinol Metab 1995; 80: 1584–90.

25. Jacqueminet S, Briaud I, Rouault C, Reach G, Poitout V. Inhibition of insulin gene expression by long-term exposure of pancreatic β-cells to palmitate is dependent on the presence of a stimulatory glucose concentration. Metabolism 2000; 49: 532–6.

26. Lupi R, Dotta F, Marselli L et al. Prolonged exposure to free fatty acids has cytostatic and pro-apoptotic effects on human pancreatic islets: evidence that β-cell death is caspase mediated, partially dependent on ceramide pathway, and Bcl-2 regulated. Diabetes 2002; 51: 1437–42.

27. Prentki M, Corkey BE. Are the β-cell signaling molecules malonyl-CoA and cytosolic long-chain acyl-CoA implicated in multiple tissue defects of obesity and NIDDM? Diabetes 1996; 45: 273–83.

28. Bakris GL, Smith AC, Richardson DJ et al. Impact of an ACE inhibitor and calcium antagonist on microalbuminuria and lipid subfractions in type 2 diabetes: a randomised, multi-centre pilot study. J Hum Hypertens 2002; 16(3): 185–91.

29. Cheung R, Lewanczuk RZ, Rodger NW et al. The effect of valsartan and captopril on lipid parameters in patients with type II diabetes mellitus and nephropathy. Int J Clin Pract 1999; 53(8): 584–92.

30. Schlueter W, Keilani T, Batlle DC. Metabolic effects of converting enzyme inhibitors: focus on the reduction of cholesterol and lipoprotein(a) by fosinopril. Am J Cardiol 1993; 72(20): 37H–44H.

31. de Zeeuw D, Remuzzi G, Parving HH et al. Proteinuria, a target for renoprotection in patients with type 2 diabetic nephropathy: lessons from RENAAL. Kidney Int 2004; 65(6): 2309–20.

32. National Heart, Lung, and Blood Institute/National Institute of Diabetes and Digestive and Kidney Diseases. Clinical Guidelines on the Identification, Evaluation, and Treatment of Overweight and Obesity in Adults. National Heart, Lung and Blood Institute, June 1998.

33. Mooradian AD, Chehade J, Thurman JE. The role of thiazolidinediones in the treatment of patients with type 2 diabetes mellitus. Treat Endocrinol 2002; 1(1): 13–20.

34. Trovati M, Cavalot F. Optimization of hypolipidemic and antiplatelet treatment in the diabetic patient with renal disease. J Am Soc Nephrol 2004; 15 (Suppl 1): S12–S20.

35. Bloomfield Rubins H, Robins SJ, Collins D et al. Diabetes, plasma insulin, and cardiovascular disease: subgroup analysis from the Department of Veterans Affairs high-density lipoprotein intervention trial (VA-HIT). Arch Intern Med 2002; 162: 2597–604.

36. Diabetes Atherosclerosis Intervention Study Investigators. Effect of fenofibrate on progression of coronary-artery disease in type 2 diabetes: the Diabetes Atherosclerosis Intervention Study, a randomised study. Lancet 2001; 357: 905–10.

37. Koskinen P, Manttari M, Manninen V et al. Coronary heart disease incidence in NIDDM patients in the Helsinki Heart Study. Diabetes Care 1992; 15: 820–5.

38. Massy ZA, Ma JZ, Louis TA, Kasiske BL. Lipid lowering therapy in patients with renal disease. Kidney Int 1995; 48: 188–98.

39. Pyörälä K, Pedersen TR, Kjekshus J et al. Cholesterol lowering with simvastatin improves prognosis of diabetic patients with coronary heart disease. A subgroup analysis of the Scandinavian Simvastatin Survival Study (4S). Diabetes Care 1997; 20: 614–20.

40. Goldberg RB, Mellies MJ, Sacks FM et al. Cardiovascular events and their reduction with pravastatin in diabetic and glucose-intolerant myocardial infarction survivors with average cholesterol levels: subgroup analyses in the cholesterol and recurrent events (CARE) trial. The Care Investigators. Circulation 1998; 98: 2513–19.

41. Heart Protection Study Collaborative Group. MRC/BHF Heart Protection Study of cholesterol-lowering with simvastatin in 5963 people with diabetes: a randomised placebo-controlled trial. Lancet 2003; 361: 2005–16.

141

42. Rosenson RS. Cholesterol lowering in diabetes. New evidence supports aggressive LDL-C targets. Postgrad Med. 2005; 117(4): 17–20, 23–7.

43. Colhoun HM, Betteridge DJ, Durrington PN et al. for the CARDS investigators. Primary prevention of cardiovascular disease with atorvastatin in type 2 diabetes in the Collaborative Atorvastatin Diabetes Study (CARDS): multicentre randomised placebo-controlled trial. Lancet 2004; 364: 685–96.

44. Stem RH, Yang BB, Horton M et al. Renal dysfunction does not alter the pharmacokinetics of LDL-cholesterol reduction of atorvastatin. J Clin Pharmacol 1997; 37: 816–19.

Case 28

A PATIENT WITH PERIPHERAL ARTERIAL DISEASE AND METABOLIC SYNDROME

Evangelos A Zacharis and Emmanuel S Ganotakis

History and examination

A 54-year-old priest was referred to the lipid clinic by a vascular surgeon, because of dyslipidemia. He had been diagnosed with intermittent claudication 2 years previously (bilateral calf discomfort while walking about 1000 m). At that time he stopped smoking (ex-smoker: 60 pack/years) and gained approximately 10 kg. He drank a glass of red wine every night. Apart from his claudication he had been in good health with no serious illness. His father died aged 60 of coronary heart disease (CHD), his mother had type 2 diabetes mellitus and his brother had CHD (PTCA + stent). The patient's medication included aspirin (100 mg/day).

On examination, his blood pressure (BP) was 140/85 mm Hg, his body mass index (BMI) was 27.2 kg/m², and his waist circumference was 105 cm. He had no stigmata of hyperlipidemia and no bruits but palpable foot pulses were absent in both legs.

Laboratory blood tests: fasting plasma glucose 100 mg/dl (5.6 mmol/l) [reference range 70–110 mg/dl (3.9–6.2 mmol/l)], urea 40 mg/dl (6.6 mmol/l) [15–55 mg/dl (2.5–9.1 mmol/l)], creatinine 0.9 mg/dl (80 μmol/l) [0.7–1.3 mg/dl (62–115 μmol/l)], alanine aminotranferase (ALT) 71 U/l [5–40 U/l], alkaline phosphatase 57 U/I [35–125 U/I], gamma glutamyl aminotransferase 20 U/l [10–75 U/l], urate 6.1 mg/dl (0.36 mmol/l) [3–7 mg/dl (0.2–0.4 mmol/l)], and plasma fibrinogen 460 mg/dl [200–400 mg/dl]. His fasting lipid profile was: total cholesterol 263 mg/dl (6.8 mmol/l), HDL-cholesterol 28 mg/dl (0.7 mmol/l), and triglycerides 500 mg/dl (5.65 mmol/l). No secondary cause of his dyslipidemia was found (thyroid function tests and oral glucose tolerance test were in the normal range).

His resting ECG was normal; the ankle-brachial index (ABI) was 0.60. Because of his peripheral arterial disease (PAD), he underwent myocardial perfusion single-photon emission computed tomography (SPECT) Th²⁰¹ with dipyridamole.

This revealed an inferior wall perfusion defect. Coronary angiography did not show any clinically significant stenosis.

Management

This 54-year-old dyslipidemic man has the metabolic syndrome (three of five diagnostic features: low HDL-cholesterol, hypertriglyceridemia, and borderline BP) according to the National Cholesterol Education Program Adult Panel III (NCEP ATP III) (2001).[1] Furthermore, PAD is characterized as a CHD equivalent in the NCEP ATP III. Patients with established CHD or a CHD equivalent should be treated with lipid-lowering drugs and the LDL-cholesterol goal level should be < 100 mg/dl (2.6 mmol/l).[1]

Another issue to be addressed is his low HDL-cholesterol. Low HDL-cholesterol is recognized as a strong independent predictor of CHD. The NCEP ATP III guidelines[1] do not specify a goal for HDL-cholesterol but they define a level below 40 mg/dl (1.0 mmol/l) as being associated with increased risk. The European guidelines (2003) make a similar statement.[2]

His very high triglyceride levels also require attention. For persons with very high triglyceride levels, the initial aim of therapy is to prevent acute pancreatitis. This includes reducing triglyceride levels pharmacologically. The NCEP ATP III[1] recommends very-low-fat diets, increased physical activity, and fibrate or nicotinic acid. At triglyceride levels > 500 mg/dl (5.65 mmol/l) the NCEP ATP III[1] states that controlling the hypertriglyceridemia is the priority of treatment.

Treatment options

(a) *Therapeutic lifestyle changes (TLC)*: include very-low-fat diets (≤ 15% of calorie intake), exercise, and weight reduction. This approach is useful in patients with mixed hyperlipidemia but may not be adequate to reach NCEP ATP III goals.[1]

(b) *Fibrates*: mainly affect triglyceride levels (reduced by 20–50%). They also have a favorable effect on HDL-cholesterol (increased by 10–25%) and a minor effect on LDL-cholesterol (reduction 5–25%). Moreover, fibrates reduce fibrinogen levels, a predictor of vascular risk and outcome.[3]

(c) *Statins*: are first-line drugs for LDL-cholesterol reduction. They reduce LDL-cholesterol by 18–55%. They can also lower triglyceride levels in a dose-dependent manner by 7–30% and raise HDL-cholesterol about 5%. The

144

Table 1 Fasting laboratory values before and after treatment

Parameter	First visit	8 weeks after starting micronized fenofibrate 200 mg/day	3 months after adding atorvastatin (40 mg/day) to micronized fenofibrate
Total cholesterol mg/dl (mmol/l)	263 (6.8)	240 (6.2)	163 (4.2)
Triglycerides mg/dl (mmol/l)	500 (5.65)	275 (3.1)	178 (2.0)
HDL-cholesterol mg/dl (mmol/l)	28 (0.7)	32 (0.8)	35 (0.9)
LDL-cholesterol mg/dl (mmol/l)	–	153 (4.0)	92 (2.4)
ALT (U/l)	54	71	40
CK (U/l)	93	88	117

ALT, alanine aminotransferase (upper limit of reference range: 40 U/l);
CK, creatine kinase (upper limit of reference range: 220 U/l).

   triglyceride-lowering effect is more pronounced when pretreatment levels are
   raised.
(d) *Combination (statin + fibrate) therapy*: this is the most comprehensive
   approach for patients with mixed dyslipidemia but it needs careful
   monitoring because of the increased risk for adverse effects. Several
   trials assessed the efficacy and safety of combination therapy.[4] In a study of
   120 patients with type 2 diabetes mellitus and combined hyperlipidemia the
   group on combination therapy (atorvastatin 20 mg + micronized fenofibrate
   200 mg) had significantly better changes in lipid values than those on
   monotherapy.[5]

   We prescribed micronized fenofibrate (200 mg/day) together with TLC. Eight
weeks later the patient was doing well. Triglycerides dropped to 275 mg/dl
(3.1 mmol/l), representing a 45% decrease from the baseline value; HDL-
cholesterol increased to 32 mg/dl (0.8 mmol/l), a rise of 14.3%. The calculated
LDL-cholesterol was 153 mg/dl (4.0 mmol/l) and we added atorvastatin
40 mg/day to improve this value. Three months later the patient was
asymptomatic with LDL-cholesterol 92 mg/dl (2.4 mmol/l) and HDL-cholesterol
35 mg/dl (0.9 mmol/l). Creative kinase (CK) and ALT levels were normal at 117
and 40 U/l, respectively (Table 1).

145

Comments

Patients with PAD are at high risk for cardiovascular events; therefore, they need aggressive risk factor modification. For patients with mixed dyslipidemia, combination therapy (statin + fibrate) with careful monitoring can provide comprehensive management of all the lipid abnormalities.

References

1. Executive Summary of the Third Report of the National Cholesterol Education Program (NCEP) Expert Panel on Detection, Evaluation, and Treatment of High Blood Cholesterol in adults (Adult Treatment Panel III). JAMA 2001; 285: 2486–97.

2. European guidelines on cardiovascular disease prevention in clinical practice. Third Joint Task Force of European and other Societies on cardiovascular disease prevention in clinical practice. *Eur J Cardiovasc Prev Rehabil* 2003; 10: S1–S10.

3. Mikhailidis DP, Ganotakis ES, Spyropoulos KA et al. Prothrombotic and lipoprotein variables in patients attending a cardiovascular risk management clinic: response to ciprofibrate or lifestyle advice. *Int Angiol* 1998; 17: 225–33.

4. Xydakis AM, Ballantyne CM. Combination therapy for combined dyslipidemia. *Am J Cardiol* 2002; 90(Suppl): 21K–29K.

5. Athyros VG, Papageorgiou AA, Athyrou VV, Demitriadis DS, Kontopoulos AG. Atorvastatin and micronized fenofibrate alone and in combination in type 2 diabetes with combined hyperlipidemia. *Diabetes Care* 2002; 25: 1198–202.

Case 29

A POSTMENOPAUSAL WOMAN WITH MARKED HYPERTRIGLYCERIDEMIA

Savitha Subramanian and Alan Chait

A 52-year-old postmenopausal woman presented with new-onset skin rash on her elbows of 4 weeks duration. One year before presentation, she was found to have mild hypertension and was started on hydrochlorothiazide. Her blood pressure was well controlled on her current dose. She had recently noted occasional mild upper abdominal discomfort, but was otherwise well. She noted vast improvement of hot flashes after starting low-dose estrogen therapy about 3 months ago. She denied any other complaints.

She reported eating a healthy diet; she exercised infrequently and had gained about 8 kg in the past 3 years. She drank two glasses of red wine every day with dinner. She had 15 pack-years of smoking but quit 5 years ago. Her family history was significant for her father, aged 70 with hypercholesterolemia, treated with atorvastatin. He was diagnosed with a myocardial infarction at age 47 and underwent coronary angioplasty and subsequently three-vessel coronary artery bypass grafting at the age of 60. Her mother, aged 68, was healthy. She has three brothers, all healthy, whose lipid levels were unknown. Her paternal grandfather died in his sleep at the age of 55. She had a paternal uncle who died of coronary disease at age 71 and another paternal uncle aged 70 who had high triglycerides.

Physical examination revealed an overweight Caucasian woman. Her blood pressure was 130/82 mm Hg. Her body mass index (BMI) was 27.9 kg/m^2. Fundus appeared pale-pink on examination. Small yellow nontender papular lesions with erythematous base were seen on her elbows as well as the buttock region. She had no other skin eruptions. Her heart sounds were normal and her lungs were clear to auscultation. Waist circumference was 95 cm. The liver was enlarged 1 cm below the right costal margin and tender to palpation. The rest of the examination was unrevealing. A fasting lipid profile revealed cholesterol of 6.7 mmol/l (normal < 5.2); triglycerides 48.6 mmol/l (normal < 1.7); HDL-cholesterol 0.65 mmol/l (normal > 1.0). The blood sample was reported as lipemic. Serum amylase and lipase, liver enzymes, creatinine, and thyroid stimulating hormone levels were all within normal range. Fasting blood glucose was 6.4 mmol/l.

147

Discussion

Marked hypertriglyceridemia is due to the presence of chylomicron particles in the circulation. Chylomicronemia refers to the presence of large lipoprotein particles in fasting plasma. 'Chylomicronemia syndrome' is defined as the presence of one or more of a set of symptoms or signs occurring in a patient with plasma triglyceride levels ≥ 22.6 mmol/l. The plasma appears turbid due to scattering of light by the large triglyceride-containing particles.

Causes

Genetic disorders of chylomicronemia are exceedingly rare and include familial lipoprotein lipase deficiency and apoC-II deficiency, both of which are autosomal recessive disorders.

The most common conditions leading to marked hypertriglyceridemia are the coexistence of one or more secondary causes of hypertriglyceridemia in conjunction with a common genetic form of hypertriglyceridemia such as familial hypertriglyceridemia or familial combined hyperlipidemia (see Box 1). In the absence of secondary causes, these two genetic forms of hyperlipidemia do not cause marked hypertriglyceridemia. When there are secondary factors present (estrogen, thiazide diuretic, and alcohol consumption in our patient), underlying genetic causes of mild triglyceride elevations lead to marked hypertriglyceridemia. The presence of a strong family history of premature vascular disease suggests that familial combined hyperlipidemia is most likely the underlying genetic cause resulting in marked triglyceride elevation.

Clinical manifestations

Symptoms and signs may occur variably in patients with marked hypertriglyceridemia. Massive hypertriglyceridemia, with triglyceride levels up to 339 mmol/l (30 000 mg/dl) can occur with no symptoms or signs. The reasons for this are unknown. However, these patients are at risk for the development of pancreatitis. Recognition and treatment of abdominal pain as part of the chylomicronemia syndrome leads to reduction in morbidity and mortality in these patients. The clinical features of chylomicronemia-associated pancreatitis are indistinguishable from that due to other causes. Hepatomegaly and less commonly

---

Box 1   Secondary causes of hypertriglyceridemia

Diabetes mellitus

Hypothyroidism

Nephrotic syndrome

Uremia/dialysis

Obesity

Alcohol

Lipodystrophy

Drugs – Diuretics (thiazides and loop)

   Beta-blockers (nonselective)

   Estrogens

   Tamoxifen

   Glucocorticoids

   Ticlopidine

   Retinoids

   Interferons – interferon-α

   Atypical antipsychotics (clozapine, olanzapine)

   Lipid infusions – total parenteral nutrition, propofol (infused as a soybean oil emulsion)

   Immunosuppressant therapy for organ transplantation (tacrolimus, sirolimus, cyclosporine)

Rare – Cushing's syndrome

   Acromegaly

   Addison's disease

   Systemic lupus erythematosus

   Glycogen storage disease type 1

Adapted from Chait and Brunzell[1] and Donahoo et al.[2]

---

splenomegaly may be noted. A thorough examination of the skin often reveals eruptive xanthomas localized over the buttocks, knees, and extensor surfaces of the arms. In this patient, the skin rashes she described were cutaneous eruptive xanthomas over the elbows. Occasionally, xanthomas may be localized only over the buttock region and can therefore be missed without complete skin examination. Eruptive xanthomas are lipid deposits in the skin that result from phagocytosis of chylomicrons by skin macrophages.

Lipemia retinalis is a characteristic appearance of the fundus of the eye with marked triglyceride elevations. The fundus and retinal arterioles and venules appear pale pink in color due to the scattering of light by the large chylomicron particles in the blood, with an exaggerated light reflex. This change is reversible, and vision is not affected. However, this is more commonly a retrospective clinical finding detected with the knowledge of existing hypertriglyceridemia, and seldom leads to a new diagnosis.

Management

The first goal in the management of patients with marked hypertriglyceridemia is to prevent acute pancreatitis. This is achieved by lowering triglyceride levels to below 11.3 mmol/l (1000 mg/dl). Acute hemorrhagic pancreatitis is the most important, life-threatening clinical consequence of chronic chylomicronemia. Chylomicron-induced pancreatitis is similar to other forms of pancreatitis and treatment includes bowel rest and nothing by mouth, moderate caloric restriction and total parenteral nutrition without lipid emulsion. Mild epigastric discomfort, as experienced by this patient, occurs with no clinical symptoms or signs of pancreatitis and is due to stretching of the liver capsule due to a fatty liver. A diet low in fat (< 10% calories from fat) should be advised until the triglyceride levels fall to levels below 11.3 mmol/l, when the risk of pancreatitis is very low.

The mainstay of treatment involves the use of drugs to specifically lower triglyceride levels. The fibric acid derivatives are effective triglyceride-lowering agents. Gemfibrozil and fenofibrate are widely used in the United States; bezafibrate and ciprofibrate are available in Europe. Niacin is another alternative which can be used for triglyceride lowering, if glucose levels are normal. This patient was started on micronized fenofibrate 145 mg once a day and, with the help of a nutritionist, she was advised to adhere to a low-fat diet. Niacin was not considered in this patient due to elevated plasma glucose levels.

Treatment of secondary causes. This patient was on a thiazide diuretic for mild hypertension and had recently started estrogen replacement therapy for vasomotor symptoms of menopause. These two drugs can cause marked hypertriglyceridemia in patients who are predisposed. Selecting a lipid-neutral antihypertensive agent such as angiotensin converting enzyme (ACE) inhibitors, angiotensin receptor blockers, calcium channel blockers or alpha-adrenergic blockers is preferred. If symptoms dictate the need for hormone replacement therapy, transdermal administration of estrogen avoids the hepatic first-pass effect and does not cause the triglyceride elevations seen with oral preparations. In this patient, estrogen was discontinued; hydrochlorothiazide was replaced with lisinopril. She was advised to avoid alcohol, since even small amounts can raise plasma triglyceride levels. These measures resulted in successful triglyceride lowering.

Cutaneous eruptive xanthomata regress with medical therapy to lower plasma triglyceride levels, therefore surgical removal is not indicated. This patient's cutaneous eruptive xanthomata completely resolved 3 months after starting therapy.

A repeat lipid profile, obtained after 3 months of therapy with fenofibrate, showed a total cholesterol of 7.2 mmol/l, triglyceride 4.8 mmol/l, LDL-cholesterol 4.9 mmol/l. The presence of high LDL levels after initiating fibrate therapy supports the diagnosis of familial combined hyperlipidemia. For primary prevention of cardiovascular events, she was started on an HMG-CoA inhibitor (statin) with good lowering of her LDL and has continued to do well with lifestyle modification and statin–fibrate combination therapy.

References

1. Chait A, Brunzell JD. Chylomicronemia syndrome. Adv Intern Med. 1992; 37: 249–73.
2. Donahoo WT, Kosmiski LA, Eckel RL. Drugs causing dyslipoproteinemia. Endocrinol Metab Clin North Am 1998; 27(3): 677–97.
3. Brunzell JD, Deeb S. In: Scriver CR, Beaudet AR, Sly WS et al., eds. The Metabolic and Molecular Basis of Inherited Disease, 8th edn. McGraw Hill, 2001: 2789–816.

Case 30

COMBINATION THERAPY OF HYPERLIPIDEMIA

Henry N Ginsberg

Introduction

At the present time, we are fortunate to have many treatments for hyperlipidemia/dyslipidemia. In the case of severe hypercholesterolemia, which is usually associated with very high levels of LDL-cholesterol in the setting of familial hypercholesterolemia, the HMG-CoA reductase inhibitors, or statins, provide a powerful and safe first line of therapy, with the ability to lower LDL-cholesterol levels between 30 and 50%. When further LDL lowering is required in these patients, bile acid binding resins, niacin, and fibrates can all add efficacy, as can ezetimibe, an inhibitor of cholesterol absorption. Niacin and fibrates, in combination with statins, may slightly increase the risk of myositis, which is about 1/2000 for statin monotherapy, but that risk is often worth taking in patients with very high risk for first or recurrent coronary artery events. In patients with combined hyperlipidemia, where both triglycerides and LDL-cholesterol levels are increased, statin therapy may still be first-line treatment when LDL-cholesterol is significantly elevated relative to the risk category of the patient, but niacin and fibrates may play a more important role here. Again, the potential for myositis must be taken into account when a therapeutic program is planned. In patients with insulin resistance/type 2 diabetes, the need for combined lipid-altering therapy may be a high priority because of the presence of severe cardiovascular disease, even when the LDL-cholesterol is not 'high'. Finally, combined treatment with niacin and fibrate may be very useful for severe hypertriglyceridemia or severely reduced HDL-cholesterol levels.

Case studies

Case 1. A 47-year-old woman comes to your office for a routine physical examination; she has not seen a doctor in several years but thinks she may have diabetes. Her previous medical history is informative for a 'touch of diabetes' during her second pregnancy, weight gain of 30 lbs during the past 10 years, and recent fatigue. Her menstrual cycle has recently become erratic and she has had a few 'hot flashes'. She has no history of visual or renal problems, and has had no symptoms of cardiovascular disease. Here family history is positive for type 2 diabetes mellitus in her mother and a maternal aunt. Her father died of a myocardial infarction at the age of 63 years.

Physical exam reveals a moderately obese women, 5'4" tall, weighing 165 lbs. Pulse is 72/min, blood pressure 140/90, respirations 16/min. Fundiscopic exam shows a few exudates and mild arteriolar narrowing. Thyroid is 20 g. Examination of the cardiovascular system reveals normal carotid pulses without bruits, normal sinus rhythm without murmers or gallops, normal femoral pulses without bruits but diminished dorsalis pedis pulses. Laboratory results include a fasting blood glucose of 110 mg/dl and a blood urea nitrogen (BUN) of 24 mg/dl. Her fasting lipid profile includes a total cholesterol of 225 mg/dl, triglycerides 250 mg/dl, HDL-cholesterol 41 mg/dl, LDL-cholesterol 134 mg/dl.

Questions:

1. What other laboratory tests would you carry out to evaluate this patient?
2. What are the therapies that will likely be necessary to minimize this patient's risk of complications?

Case 2. A 37-year-old female is referred because of severe hypercholesterolemia present even after initiation of therapy with an HMG-CoA reductase inhibitor. Her family history is positive for severe hypercholesterolemia (>400 mg/dl) in her paternal grandmother, who died from a myocardial infarction at the age of 60 years, and her father, who had a coronary artery bypass graft (CABG) at age 45 years. The patient has been in general good health, and exercises four or five times per week, running and biking. She eats a low-fat diet, this began in childhood, and has never smoked. She is married with three children, who all have normal cholesterol levels, and has had bilateral tubal ligations. She is still menstruating regularly.

On physical exam, she appears well except for xanthelasma and xanthomas over her metacarpal joints, below the knees, and on her Achilles tendons. She has a 1/6 systolic ejection murmer. The rest of her exam is normal. Medications include atorvastatin, 10 mg daily, and multivitamins. Laboratory exam reveals a total cholesterol of 230 mg/dl, triglyceride 75 mg/dl, HDL-cholesterol 55 mg/dl, and LDL-cholesterol 200 mg/dl. All other lab tests are normal.

Questions:

1. What other laboratory tests should you conduct to fully evaluate this patient's risk for complications of diabetes mellitus?
2. What are the therapies that will likely be necessary to minimize this patient's risk of complications?

154

Recommended reading

Ginsberg HN. Insulin resistance and cardiovascular disease. J Clin Invest 2000; 106: 453–8.

Ginsberg HN. Hypertriglyceridemia: new insights and new approaches to treatment. Am J Cardiol 2001; 87: 1174–80.

Ginsberg HN, Goldberg IJ. Disorders of lipoprotein metabolism. In: Fauci AS, et al., eds. Harrison's Principles of Internal Medicine, 14th edn. New York: McGraw Hill, 1998.

Ginsberg HN, Tuck C. Diabetes and dyslipidemia. In: Johnstone MT, Veves A, eds. Diabetes and Cardiovascular Disease. Towata, NJ: Humana Press, 2001.

Horowitz B, Ginsberg HN. Evaluation and treatment of dyslipidemia in diabetes mellitus. In: DeFronzo RA, ed. Current Management of Diabetes Mellitus. Philadelphia, PA: Mosby-Year Book, 1997.

Answers

Case 1. This woman presents many of the features of 'syndrome X' or the 'metabolic syndrome'; the cluster of diabetes, dyslipidemia, hypertension, and obesity. This complex phenotype is linked to insulin resistance, which is possibly the central pathophysiologic feature. Her past history of gestational glucose intolerance or diabetes is compatible with the long prediabetic period before the onset of hyperglycemia, with elevations of plasma glucose during periods of stress or hormonal alterations. Her family history is typical for the dominant transmission of type 2 diabetes. Probably most important is her weight gain during the previous decade, leading to increased insulin resistance and possible loss of insulin secretory capacity.

Additional laboratory tests should include HbA1c to assess whether her plasma glucose is consistently high postprandially, and a 24-hour urine collection to evaluate protein excretion and creatinine clearance. The latter is crucial because of her hypertension, elevated BUN, and the association of proteinuria with cardiovascular mortality in individuals with the insulin resistance syndrome. Additionally, even moderate proteinuria is associated with alterations in plasma lipid levels; in particular hypertriglyceridemia and low HDL-cholesterol. Lipoprotein (a) should be measured as well because it is elevated in the presence of microalbuminuria. Other measurements that would be of academic interest, but without therapeutic relevance at this time would include apoprotein B, homocysteine, insulin, LDL size, and C-reactive protein.

This is a patient at very high risk for macrovascular complications: she has the insulin resistance syndrome with hypertension and mild dyslipidemia. She is also

155

entering menopause. The first approach to this patient should be diet, exercise, and weight loss. At this stage of her diabetes, and considering her plasma glucose level, she might be able to normalize glucose levels with significant weight reduction, dietary modification and exercise. The optimal diet, in view of her high risk for arteriosclerotic cardiovascular disease (ASCVD), would be a diet low in saturated fat, cholesterol, and calories. Although it would be nice to simply take saturated fats out of the diet and not replace them, it is more likely that some replacement will be needed, at least at a later time. There is controversy as to whether carbohydrates or monounsaturated fats (and possibly polyunsaturated fats) should be used as replacement calories for saturated fats. One must balance the somewhat lower triglycerides and slightly higher HDL-cholesterol that are achieved when monounsaturates, rather than carbohydrates, are used to replace saturated fats, with the greater risk of increased weight when someone eats a higher fat diet. Of importance is the finding that simply using complex carbohydrates (starches) versus simple sugars does not really affect plasma glucose, insulin or triglyceride levels; patients must eat carbohydrate foods that are high in fiber to maintain lower glucose and triglyceride levels all day long.

The question of drug treatment in this patient is complex. When should diet and exercise be abandoned as sole therapy? The answer to this question will have to be based on individual aspects of the case and the wishes of the patient and possibly the physician. In terms of risk for ASCVD, the goal of any therapy, including treatment to lower glucose concentrations, would be to optimize lipid levels. This patient's LDL is above the goal of 130 mg/dl recommended for someone with two or more risk factors. The low saturated fat, low cholesterol diet (AHA Step 2 diet) that will be prescribed could lower her LDL about 10%, bringing her close to 130 mg/dl. The decision to treat with specific lipid-altering therapy would depend on changes achieved with diet, exercise, and potential glucose-lowering treatment. Although her dyslipidemia at presentation indicates that significant improvement in triglycerides and possibly HDL will be achieved with diet, exercise, and weight loss, her very high-risk profile for ASCVD suggests that more aggressive LDL therapy, such as that achieved with a HMG-CoA reductase inhibitor, would be beneficial. If her LDL-cholesterol was lowered to about 100 mg/dl without much change in triglycerides and HDL, the issue of combination therapy – with the addition of either niacin or a fibrate to the statin – could be considered. Certainly, the overall lipid profile would improve on either combination, but the risk of side effects would increase. The most significant risk would be from myositis, with potential for rhabdomyolysis, myoglobinemia, and renal dysfunction. However, the literature shows that the risk of myositis is only about 1% in clinical trials of statins and fibrates, and the risk with fenofibrate may be less than with gemfibrozil. The risk of myositis during treatment with statins and niacin is probably much less than 1%. Hormone replacement therapy would

156

probably lower LDL- and raise HDL-cholesterol levels, but recent studies indicate that such therapy will not provide benefit in terms of cardiovascular disease. Indeed, combined estrogen and progestin therapy may be associated with increased risk for vascular events. Additionally, hormone replacement therapy will, however, increase plasma triglyceride levels, and this can be extreme in some cases, even with the development of pancreatitis.

Case 2. This patient clearly has fairly severe familial hypercholesterolemia (FH), with an estimated level of untreated LDL-cholesterol of over 300 mg/dl, xanthomas, and a poor family history. It would be important to determine what her LDL-cholesterol was before any treatment so that we could rule out a lack of response. But barring that possibility, what should be done next?

Other laboratory measures could include a TSH level (unlikely to be playing a role but worth the look). A homocysteine level would give more risk information but she should be on a multivitamin in any event. There is the possibility that she has a high level of lipoprotein (a); her father's early disease, even in the face of FH, suggests a concomitant high lipoprotein (a) level and if this was identified, it would increase the need for aggressive LDL-lowering therapy. C-reactive protein would be interesting but it is not clear what it would mean for treatment. Should this patient have a stress ECG test – she exercises regularly without signs. Should she have an electron beam computed tomography (EBCT) to determine if significant coronary artery calcium exists at this date – her systolic murmer could be indicative of aortic valve calcification.

As for treatment, she definitely needs her LDL-cholesterol lowered further. Initial treatment would include titration of her statin to full dose of 80 mg/dl; this would be expected to lower her LDL about 18% (three doublings of the dose) to a level of about 170 mg/dl. Addition of a bile acid binding resin is safe and effective; statins and resins are synergistic and one might get an additional 20% lowering with a modest dose of the first generation resins or with a full dose of colesevalem. The recent availability of ezetimibe, a cholesterol absorption blocker, offers physicians another tool for LDL lowering, with 10 mg ezetimibe giving 15–20% LDL lowering. If her LDL was then at 130–140 mg/dl, the decision to stop or continue with either niacin or a fibrate would depend on the other laboratory findings.

Case 31

Use Of Combination Therapy In A Patient With Complex Dyslipidemia

Peter P Toth and Michael H Davidson

Introduction

The dyslipidemias are a highly heterogeneous class of metabolic disorders that can give rise to a wide range of diseases. A variety of congenital enzymopathies, mutations in cell surface receptors, and derangements in apoprotein function can predispose to abnormalities in circulating lipoprotein concentrations. Dyslipidemia is a pivotal risk factor for the development of atherosclerosis and its various clinical sequelae, including myocardial infarction, sudden death, ischemic stroke, and peripheral vascular disease. Elevations in LDL-cholesterol and triglyceride are associated with increased risk for cardiovascular disease (CVD), while high serum levels of HDL-cholesterol are associated with reduced risk for CVD.

In recent years a number of drug classes have been developed in an effort to modulate the absorption, production, and distribution of cholesterol and triglycerides.[1] Prospective clinical outcome trials in both the primary and secondary prevention settings continue to substantiate the important role that lipid management plays in reducing risk for CVD in patients with dyslipidemia. The case presented herein examines the importance of combination therapy when all components of the lipid profile are abnormal and single agent therapy alone cannot facilitate achievement of guideline-specified goals.

The case

HS is a 57-year-old Caucasian male who has undergone multivessel coronary artery bypass grafting for coronary artery disease (CAD) in his proximal left main, mid circumflex, and proximal right coronary arteries. Three years subsequent to his bypass surgery the internal mammary graft to his left main vessel required stenting. Since this stenting procedure he has had no angina. He has required a right-sided carotid endarterectomy following an ischemic cerebrovascular accident which left him with some left lower extremity weakness, although he remains ambulatory. He currently has a 20% occlusion along the carotid bifurcation on the left side. He has no history of claudication and has brisk peripheral pulses. He does not smoke. The patient has been diabetic for 20 years. His HbA1c 1 month ago was 8.0%. He is currently on metformin 1000 mg po bid and glipizide 5 mg po bid. He has no history of diabetic nephropathy and does not have nephrotic syndrome. He has well controlled hypertension (blood pressure sitting 121/76 mm Hg) for which he is taking ramipril 10 mg po qd, metoprolol 50 mg po bid, and hydrochlorothiazide 12.5 mg po qd. The liver function panel with transaminase levels is normal. Serum TSH is 2.32. HS does not drink alcohol due to religious beliefs and he is not taking any type of antipsychotic medication that might impact triglyceride levels. HS is quite obese with a body mass index (BMI) of 41. He has failed multiple supervised attempts at weight loss through increased physical activity and reduced caloric intake.

He is referred to the lipid clinic because of a very challenging lipid profile. He quite appropriately was already on simvastatin 40 mg po qd. His direct LDL-cholesterol is 69 mg/dl. HDL-cholesterol is 29 mg/dl, and triglycerides are 1050 mg/dl. The referring physician is concerned about two issues. First, the patient's HDL-cholesterol is very low. According to the National Cholesterol Education Program Adult Treatment Panel III, an HDL-cholesterol < 40 mg/dl constitutes an independent risk factor for CAD and therapeutic effort should be expended to raise the HDL-cholesterol.[2] After careful counseling about how to take the medication, she has tried to treat him with low doses of niacin and then Niaspan, but after some episodes of flushing, he refuses to try either formulation again. Second, the patient's triglycerides are markedly elevated. Not only do they constitute a risk factor for CAD, but triglycerides this high also leave the patient vulnerable to the development of pancreatitis. There could be no reasonable expectation that simply doubling the dosage of simvastatin to 80 mg would normalize this patient's serum triglycerides and HDL-cholesterol.

The referring physician's concerns are well substantiated by the literature. Although the NCEP does not offer a specific target for HDL raising, it does emphasize that trying to raise HDL-cholesterol through lifestyle modification and pharmacologic intervention is warranted in high-risk patients such as HS. The American Diabetes Association specifically endorses a target of 40 mg/dl and 50 mg/dl in male and female diabetics, respectively.[3] Raising HDL-cholesterol appears to beneficially impact risk through a number of mechanisms.[4] HDLs drive reverse cholesterol transport, a process whereby cholesterol is extracted from the

160

cellular constituents of vessel walls and delivered back to the liver for disposal as bile salts. HDLs also possess a number of anti-inflammatory, antithrombotic, and antiproliferative effects that antagonize many of the events most fundamental to atherogenesis. When triglycerides are this high, they certainly do pose a hazard for pancreatitis. Hypertriglyceridemia can arise from excess lipid absorption through the gastrointestinal tract, insulin resistance at the level of adipose tissue, impaired triglyceride catabolism in serum, or a combination of these three factors.[5]

Reducing risk for pancreatitis and optimizing the glycemic control were high clinical priorities. The patient was placed under the care of a dietitian for a palatable low-fat diet. He was also started on pioglitazone 15 mg po qd and fenofibrate 145 mg po qd. The rationale for initiating these drugs is as follows. The patient is obese and diabetic. He is manifesting evidence of insulin resistance with high triglycerides, low HDL-cholesterol, and high serum glucose, and he is hypertensive. In patients with insulin resistance, hormone-sensitive lipase in adipose tissue does not respond normally to insulin and engages in excessive hydrolysis of triglycerides stored in adipocytes, thereby releasing them into serum. Lipoprotein lipase is the enzyme in serum that hydrolyzes the triglycerides in chylomicrons and very low-density lipoproteins (VLDLs) (Figure 1). This enzyme is highly sensitive to insulin. In patients with insulin resistance, the activity of this enzyme is decreased. Pioglitazone is a thiazolidinedione (TZD) and insulin sensitizer. The thiazolidinediones help to relieve hypertriglyceridemia over the course of months as insulin sensitivity is increased. Fenofibrate drives triglyceride catabolism via a different route: these drugs decrease expression of the inhibitor of lipoprotein lipase (apoprotein CIII) and increase expression of its activator (apoprotein CII), thereby increasing activity of the enzyme. Fenofibrate is the fibrate of choice to use in combination with a statin, as gemfibrozil has a 15-fold higher risk of inducing a potentially catastrophic drug interaction (blocking statin glucuronidation), which can increase risk for rhabdomyolysis.[6]

Fibrates and TZDs also increase serum levels of HDL-cholesterol. As these drugs activate lipoprotein lipase, surface coat mass from chylomicrons and VLDL can be used to synthesize HDL in serum. A low triglyceride content in the transferred surface coat mass makes the HDL particle an unfavorable target for hepatic lipase, an enzyme that can catabolize HDL, keeping serum levels of this lipoprotein low (Figure 1). Moreover, the fibrates can directly stimulate the expression of hepatic HDL production since they are peroxisome proliferator activated receptor-α agonists.

Twelve weeks after beginning this regimen and with subsequent titration of the pioglitazone to 45 mg, the patient's lipid and liver panel were re-evaluated. The liver functions remained normal and the patient was not experiencing any myalgias, proximal weakness, nausea, or other adverse events. The patient's HbA1c improved to 6.9%. Serum LDL-cholesterol was 81 mg/dl, triglycerides

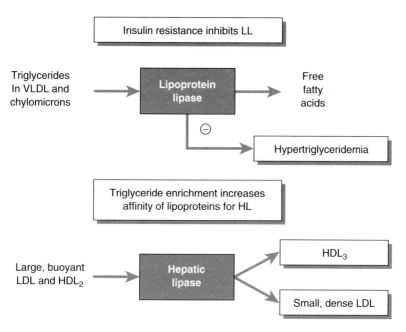

Figure 1 *Schematic depiction of lipoprotein catabolism by lipase enzymes. Lipoprotein lipase (LL) hydrolyzes the triglycerides found in the hydrophobic core of chylomicrons and very low-density lipoproteins (VLDLs) to free fatty acids and glycerol. Insulin activates this enzyme. In patients who are insulin resistant, the activity of this enzyme is reduced and the concentration of large triglyceride-enriched lipoproteins increases in serum, giving rise to hypertriglyceridemia. The fibrates can activate lipoprotein lipase by promoting the production of apoprotein CII and reducing the production of apoprotein CIII. The apoproteins constitute an activator and an inhibitor of this enzyme, respectively. In patients with high serum triglyceride levels, the LDL and HDL produced from VLDL and chylomicron metabolism yield lipoproteins enriched in triglycerides. These lipoproteins are favorable targets for another member of the lipase family of enzymes, hepatic lipase (HL). This enzyme can catabolize the large, buoyant fractions of these lipoproteins into smaller, denser lipoproteins. As LDL becomes smaller and denser it becomes relatively more atherogenic. As HDL becomes relatively smaller and denser (HDL$_3$) it becomes more prone to progressive catabolism to its constituent phospholipids and apoproteins and subsequent systemic clearance via the kidney, thereby resulting in what can be substantial reductions in serum levels of this protective lipoprotein.*

decreased to 570 mg/dl, and HDL-cholesterol increased to 41 mg/dl. His triglycerides clearly remained unacceptably high.

The patient admitted that he had difficulty adhering to some of the more stringent components of his diet. He had tried high-dose fish oils in the past but

162

found them to be 'disagreeable.' He was continued on his current pharmacologic regimen and supplemented with orlistat 120 mg with each meal. The mechanism of action of this drug as a pancreatic lipase inhibitor and the expectation of oily stools with the possibility of diarrhea were explained. The patient tolerated the drug quite well. Eight weeks after drug initiation his LDL-cholesterol was 79 mg/dl, triglycerides 168 mg/dl, and HDL-cholesterol 43 mg/dl. After 6 months of therapy with orlistat, the patient's lipid panel was maintained and he lost 16 pounds.

Conclusion

Mechanistically, this patient's case can best be explained by a partial congenital lipoprotein lipase deficiency that was exacerbated by insulin resistance. In addition to statin therapy, he required multiple adjuvant interventions with drugs that impacted the absorption, storage, and catabolism of lipid. Many dyslipidemic patients, particularly if they have metabolic syndrome and/or diabetes mellitus, will require combination therapy with lifestyle modification to achieve guideline-specified targets of all components of the lipid profile.

References

1. Davidson MH, Toth PP. Comparative effects of lipid-lowering therapies. Prog Cardiovasc Dis 2004; 47: 73–104.
2. Expert Panel on Detection, Evaluation, and Treatment of High Blood Cholesterol in Adults: Executive summary of the third report of the National Cholesterol Education Program (NCEP) Expert Panel on Detection, Evaluation, and Treatment of High Blood Cholesterol in Adults (Adult Treatment Panel III). JAMA 2001, 285: 2486–97.
3. American Diabetes Association. Dyslipidemia management in adults with diabetes. Diabetes Care 2004; 27(Suppl 1): S68–S71.
4. Toth PP. High-density lipoprotein and cardiovascular disease. Circulation 2004; 109: 1809–12.
5. Toth PP. Dyslipoproteinemias. In: Rakel RR, Bope W, eds. Conn's Current Therapy. The Netherlands: Elsevier, 2006.
6. Jones PH, Davidson MH. Reporting rate of rhabdomyolysis with fenofibrate + statin versus gemfibrozil + any statin. Am J Cardiol 2005; 95: 120–2.

Case 32

TRIPLE THERAPY IN THE TREATMENT OF HYPERLIPIDEMIA

Anthony S Wierzbicki

Introduction

Clinical trials of lipid lowering in patients with coronary heart disease (CHD) had led to ever lower targets being adopted for LDL-cholesterol and also to the recognition that raising HDL-cholesterol may be associated with benefit. This case report describes a patient with familial hypercholesterolemia (FH), hypoalphalipoproteinemia, and a high level of lipoprotein (a) who presented with an acute coronary syndrome at a young age.

Case report

A 36-year-old male presented to a local hospital with acute anterior chest pain radiating to the left arm associated with acute shortness of breath. Initial investigations rapidly established that he had an acute coronary syndrome on the basis of elevated troponin I levels and he was transferred to a teaching hospital cardiology unit for investigation. He was reviewed on the metabolic lipid round the next day.

He developed chest pain initially related to exertion at age 35 in cold weather and had been admitted to another unit with a myocardial infarction (MI) for which he had later had an elective coronary angioplasty. He had had a previous episode of severe chest pain at age 19, which he had ascribed to a football injury Since his recent admission he had been pain-free but suffered from continual tiredness and aching heavy legs. Previous family screening had established that he had a plasma cholesterol >9 mmol/l and he had been treated with simvastatin 20 mg. He had never smoked, and was teetotal. He had no drug allergies or intolerances. His only other medical history was of ankylosing spondylitis diagnosed at age 27.

The family history of cardiovascular disease was extremely strong in that his father had died of an MI at age 57 having had an initial event at age 41. His mother was fit and well. His paternal grandfather died of myocardial infarct at age 65, although he seems to have had three previous cardiac admissions. His brother, aged 33 years, had been established to have FH on the basis of total cholesterol of 12 mmol/l, and angina followed by coronary artery bypass grafting at age 26. Another brother aged 31 had hypertension and a high cholesterol sufficient to warrant statin therapy. His two eldest sons (aged 16 and 18 years) were normocholesterolemic but his other son aged 12 and daughter aged 10 had not had their lipids checked.

On examination he had thin bilateral arci and small tendon xanthomata were noticed on the second and third fingers of both hands.

His 33-year-old brother was reviewed when visiting the coronary care unit and was established to have a very similar lipid profile.

Management plan

His admission lipid profile was total cholesterol 8.3 mmol/l, triglycerides 1.55 mmol/l, HDL-cholesterol 0.88 mmol/l, and calculated LDL-cholesterol 6.5 mmol/l (Table 1). His drug therapy was altered to 80 mg atorvastatin and 10 mg ezetimibe, which improved his lipid results to total cholesterol 4.7 mmol/l, triglycerides 0.70 mmol/l, HDL-cholesterol 0.85 mmol/l, and calculated LDL-cholesterol 3.54 mmol/l. His alanine transaminase level had fallen to 49 IU/l. At review 6 weeks later these levels were not ideal for a patient at continuing high risk of cardiovascular disease, so nicotinic acid (Niaspan) was added using a titration protocol of 375 mg for 4 weeks, 500 mg for 4 weeks, 750 mg for 4 weeks increasing to the desired dose of 1 g/day in divided doses. His aspirin was made coincident with niacin and the niacin was taken with food or snacks to reduce the number of episodes of flushing. His lipid results at review 4 months later were: total cholesterol 4.4 mmol/l, triglycerides 0.78 mmol/l, HDL-cholesterol 0.91 mmol/l, and calculated LDL-cholesterol 3.04 mmol/l. He had had three episodes of flushing, all associated with consumption of curries. Although his lipid profile showed little obvious change, he was compliant with therapy and detailed density-gradient lipid and apolipoprotein ultracentrifugation established that niacin therapy had resulted in a shift of apolipoprotein A and B-100 to larger more buoyant particles.

He continues well and has had no further episodes of chest pain. He does not wish to increase his niacin further due to the unpleasant burning nature of the flushing associated with this agent.

166

Table 1 Lipid results in two brothers with familial hypercholesterolemia and early-onset coronary heart disease

Parameter	Patient initial values (simvastatin)	Patient atorvastatin–ezetimibe	Patient atorvastatin–ezetimibe–niacin	Brother initial values	Brother atorvastatin–ezetimibe–niacin
Total cholesterol (mmol/l)	8.30	4.70	4.40	9.30	4.70
Triglycerides (mmol/l)	1.50	0.70	0.78	2.25	0.79
HDL-cholesterol (mmol/l)	0.85	0.88	0.91	0.82	0.85
LDL-cholesterol (mmol/l)	6.75	3.54	3.04	7.48	3.49
ApoA-1 (g/l)	0.91	0.98	0.99	0.94	0.97
ApoB (g/l)	1.73	1.08	1.02	1.89	1.14
Lipoprotein (a) (g/l)	2.91	2.61	2.31	1.46	1.25
Glucose (mmol/l)	4.9	5.0	5.2	4.0	4.3
Insulin (pmol/l)	45	47	55	42	45
C-reactive protein (mg/l)	5.3	3.3	3.2	4.3	10
GFR (ml/min/1.73 m^2)	102	126	132	106	101

GFR, glomerular filtration rate.

167

Discussion

This case report illustrates a severe case of FH with a typical autosomal dominant inheritance pattern of both hypercholesterolemia and early-onset coronary heart disease (CHD). The severity of disease in this case was exacerbated by a number of factors including familial hypoalphalipoproteinemia, a highly elevated lipoprotein (a), raised (C-reative protein) (CRP), and a history of autoimmune disease (ankylosing spondylitis). All these factors would increase risk of cardiovascular disease.

This case illustrates a number of points. Although he had technically been treated with an evidence-based dose of simvastatin (20 mg) using data from the Scandinavian Simvastatin Survival Study, this had been insufficient to reduce his LDL-cholesterol to 3 mmol/l. Even using the advised dose of atorvastatin (80 mg), validated in the PROVE-IT study for patients with acute coronary syndromes, his lipids were unlikely to reach target as the probable extra reduction on switching statin and titrating would be 1.5 mmol/l, and therefore he required the addition of the cholesterol absorption inhibitor ezetimibe to achieve levels close to those desired for LDL-cholesterol (a 2.75 mmol/l reduction). His LDL-cholesterol levels are now within the targets set as a result of the Atorvastatin-Simvastatin Atherosclerosis Prevention (ASAP) study in patients with FH shown to prevent progression of carotid intima media thickness (cIMT).[1] His management regime follows the intervention arm in the PREVENT study that follows on from ASAPS through a randomized trial of addition of ezetimibe to maximal statin therapy in the same group using the same endpoint.

Unfortunately statin—ezetimibe therapy did not address his other risk factors including hypoalphalipoproteinemia and elevated lipoprotein (a). The addition of niacin was likely to increase his HDL-cholesterol and apolipoprotein A-1, reduce his triglycerides, deliver some extra LDL-cholesterol reduction, and reduce his lipoprotein (a). Data from both the familial atherosclerosclerosis treatment study (FATS) combining statin, niacin, and cholestyramine show that this triple therapy reduces progression of coronary atherosclerosis on quantitative angiography and events in (an underpowered) *post hoc* analysis. More recent data from the Arterial Biology for the Investigation of the Treatment Effects of Reducing Cholesterol (ARBITER)-2 study show that addition of niacin to simvastatin 40 mg reduces progression of cIMT in patients with established CHD, admittedly with far less severe hyperlipidemia, within 1 year.[2] In practice niacin therapy had little effect on HDL-cholesterol or apolipoprotein A-I levels in this family but did reduce LDL-cholesterol, apolipoprotein B, and lipoprotein (a) levels. The significance of lipoprotein (a) as a cardiovascular risk factor is unclear, as some studies fail to identify it as a risk factor for CHD and there is very poor inter-assay agreement due to problems in standardization. Its role as a risk factor was negated in FATS by

168

adequate treatment of LDL-cholesterol,[3] so there may not be a role for targeted treatment of lipoprotein (a) alone. The only current therapy for lipoprotein (a) (i.e. niacin) also had ancillary benefits on HDL and LDL particle size and distributions in this population and did reduce LDL-cholesterol further in this family.

This case illustrates the need to pursue family screening in FH aggressively and to ensure adequate treatment of their hypercholesterolemia. In families with a severe phenotype for risk of CHD measurement of ancillary risk factors may identify other lipid risk factors that require treatment. Just as in patients with hypertension, some patients may require multiple therapies to achieve reasonable control of their cardiovascular risk factors.

References

1. Smilde TJ, van Wissen S, Wollersheim H et al. Effect of aggressive versus conventional lipid lowering on atherosclerosis progression in familial hypercholesterolaemia (ASAP): a prospective, randomised, double-blind trial. Lancet 2001; 357(9256): 577–81.
2. Taylor AJ, Sullenberger LE, Lee HJ et al. Arterial Biology for the Investigation of the Treatment Effects of Reducing Cholesterol (ARBITER) 2. A double-blind, placebo-controlled study of extended-release niacin on atherosclerosis progression in secondary prevention patients treated with statins. Circulation 2004; 110: 826–34.
3. Maher VM, Brown BG, Marcovina SM et al. Effects of lowering elevated LDL cholesterol on the cardiovascular risk of lipoprotein(a). JAMA 1995; 274: 1771–4.

Case 33

GRASPING THE NETTLE: THE IMPACT OF LIFESTYLE CHANGE IN METABOLIC SYNDROME

Maria Adiseshiah and D John Betteridge

History

A 48-year-old Caucasian male was referred to cardiology with a history of dyspnea and palpitations. Thallium stress testing showed no evidence of ischemic heart disease (IHD). Total cholesterol was found to be 8.4 mmol/l. He was referred to the Lipid Clinic where the abnormal lipid profile was confirmed. Total cholesterol was 7.9 mmol/l, triglyceride 2.3, calculated LDL-cholesterol 5.85 mmol/l and HDL-cholesterol 1.0; fasting glucose was 6.1 mmol/l. Glucose intolerance had been diagnosed 2 years previously with a 2-hour post glucose load value of 8.4 mmol/l. He had stopped smoking 15 years earlier and enjoyed a moderate alcohol intake of 21 units per week. An only child, his father developed IHD in his late sixties and at the age of 74 underwent coronary artery bypass grafting. His mother is alive and well in her mid seventies. A paternal aunt is known to have diabetes mellitus.

Examination and investigations

On examination he was obese (BMI 30.5 kg/m^2). His blood pressure was 137/83 mm Hg and his pulse, heart sounds, and lung fields were normal. An early arcus was noted but no xanthomata. He described a history of left-sided chest pain. Exercise stress electrocardiography was requested and he exercised for over 10 minutes according to the Bruce protocol, attaining a maximum workload of 13.47 METS without ST changes or chest pain. Detailed biochemistry showed a high apoprotein B of 1.67 g/l and a lipoprotein (a) of 0.44 g/l (range 0–0.3 g/l).

Treatment and outcome

He was advised to lose some weight and an initial target of 90 kg was agreed. On subsequent review 6 months later he had gained 4 kg in weight, taking his weight to over 100 kg. His blood pressure was now 140/90 mm Hg. He had developed thirst and reported nocturia. Fasting blood glucose was 7.1 mmol/l.

The option of introducing metformin therapy was discussed with him. As his total cholesterol was 6.7 mmol/l with an LDL-cholesterol of 4.4 mmol/l, atorvastatin 10 mg daily was prescribed. Over the next couple of years he managed to lose weight but always regained it. Metformin therapy was introduced as his fasting blood glucose remained at 7.0 mmol/l.

Three and a half years after the initial referral he presented in clinic having lost 20 kg with diet and exercise over the previous 8 months. The effect of this weight loss on his metabolic parameters was marked. Metformin therapy had been discontinued as his fasting blood glucose had fallen to 5.8 mmol/l. Blood pressure was now 121/81 mm Hg. Total cholesterol was now 4.6 mmol/l and triglycerides 0.9 mmol/l on atorvastatin 10 mg/day. Notably his HDL-cholesterol had increased to 1.9 mmol/l and this continued to increase as weight loss and exercise levels were sustained. Latest results show a fasting blood glucose of 5.5 mmol/l, total cholesterol 5.1 mmol/l, triglycerides 0.8 mmol/l, LDL-cholesterol 2.3 mmol/l, and HDL-cholesterol 2.4 mmol/l. At 76.9 kg his BMI is now 24.5 kg/m^2.

Learning points

- In addition to hypercholesterolemia and glucose intolerance, other cardiovascular risk factors for this patient, often ignored in risk factor calculators, included obesity, family history, and a raised lipoprotein (a), recognized as a risk factor for ischemic heart disease (IHD) in the presence of a raised cholesterol.
- The risk assessment took into consideration that people who are glucose intolerant are at increased risk of cardiovascular disease compared with those with normal glycemia.
- This patient presented with marked mixed lipemia. In most patients this requires a higher dose of statin to reach therapeutic goal than in pure hypercholesterolemia. However, his lipid profile responded well to lifestyle modification and he could attain treatment goals on low dose atorvastatin.
- We know that a healthy diet coupled with regular exercise can increase HDL-cholesterol. There was considerable improvement in this patient's lipid profile with weight loss and exercise on the same low dose of statin.

In conclusion, this patient's requirement for pharmacotherapy was reduced by his lifestyle adjustments and by his success in breaking the 'yo-yo' weight cycle.

Further reading

Barter P, Kastelein J, Nunn A, Hobbs R. High-density lipoproteins (HDLs) and atherosclerosis; the unanswered questions. Atherosclerosis 2003; 168: 195–211.

Kraus WE, Houmard JA, Duscha BD et al. Effects of the amount and intensity of exercise on plasma lipoproteins. N Engl J Med 2002; 347: 1483–92.

Lehmann R, Engler H, Honegger R, Riesen W, Spinas GA. Alterations of lipolytic enzymes and high-density lipoprotein subfractions induced by physical activity in type 2 diabetes mellitus. Eur J Clin Invest 2001; 31: 37–44.

Myers J. Exercise and cardiovascular health. Circulation 2003; 107: e2–5.

NIH Consensus Conference. Physical activity and cardiovascular health. JAMA 1996; 276(3): 241–6.

Olchawa B, Kingwell BA, Hoang A et al. Physical fitness and reverse cholesterol transport. Arteriosclerosis, Thrombosis, and Vascular Biology, 2004; 24: 1087–91.

Sviridov D, Nestel P. Dynamics of reverse cholesterol transport; protection against atherosclerosis. Atherosclerosis 2002; 161: 245–54.

Thompson PD, Buchner D, Pina IL et al. Exercise and physical activity in the prevention and treatment of atherosclerotic cardiovascular disease: a statement from the Council on Clinical Cardiology (Subcommittee on Exercise, Rehabilitation, and Prevention) and the Council on Nutrition, Physical Activity, and Metabolism (Subcommittee on Physical Activity). Circulation 2003; 107: 3109–16.

Case 34

A Patient With Dyslipidemia, Coronary Heart Disease, And A History Of Statin Intolerance

Evangelos N Liberopoulos and Dimitri P Mikhailidis

History and examination

A 62-year-old man was referred with dyslipidemia and a history of myocardial infarction (MI) 9 months earlier. He had undergone percutaneous coronary intervention (PCI) with stent placement. His father had a MI at the same age and died on his way to the hospital. Furthermore, his sister was receiving lipid-lowering therapy. He had no children.

The patient's medication included: aspirin (75 mg/day), clopidogrel (75 mg/day), lansoprazole (30 mg/day), ramipril (10 mg/day), atenolol (25 mg/day), and OMACOR (concentrated omega-3 fish-oil esters, 1 g/day). He had never smoked. He had a history of hypertension and impaired glucose tolerance (IGT).

The patient had previously discontinued treatment with simvastatin, atorvastatin, and pravastatin due to muscle pain. He developed generalized symmetric muscle stiffness and aches 3 days after starting each statin. His serum creatine kinase (CK) activity had gone up to as high as 1534 U/l (upper limit of reference range = 220 U/l). Symptoms resolved about 3 days after stopping each statin and the CK returned to normal about 1 week later.

On examination, his blood pressure (BP) was 130/70 mm Hg, his waist circumference was 99 cm (39 in) and his body mass index (BMI) was 25 kg/m^2. There were no other relevant findings.

His fasting glucose was 4.8 mmol/l (87 mg/dl) but his glycated hemoglobin was 6.7% (reference range: 3.9–6.1%). His CK activity and lipid profile are shown in Table 1. Serum creatinine levels and thyroid-stimulating hormone (TSH) activity were within the reference range. Impaired renal function and/or hypothyroidism may increase the risk of statin-related muscular side effects. Hypothyroidism is also a cause of hypercholesterolemia.

175

Table 1 Fasting serum lipids and CK activity before and after treatment

Parameter	First visit	6 weeks after starting ezetimibe (10 mg/day)	2 months after adding fluvastatin (20 mg/day) to ezetimibe (10 mg/day)
Total cholesterol (mmol/l)	6.1	5.3	4.5
Triglycerides (mmol/l)	1.4	2.2	1.7
HDL-cholesterol (mmol/l)	1.3	1.2	1.2
LDL-cholesterol (mmol/l)	4.2	3.1	2.5
CK (U/l)	118	79	76

CK; creatine kinase (upper limit of reference range: 220 U/l).

Management

The patient was at high risk for subsequent vascular events since he had a previous MI plus multiple risk factors (gender, age, family history, IGT, and hypertension). Furthermore, when we first saw him his serum LDL-cholesterol was 4.1 mmol/l (158 mg/dl) (Table 1). We did not have access to his earlier laboratory values.

According to the National Cholesterol Education Program Adult Treatment Panel III (NCEP ATP III) (2004), his LDL-cholesterol goal should be < 2.6 mmol/l (100 mg/dl) with an optional level of < 1.8 mmol/l (70 mg/dl).[1] Similar goals are defined in the European (2003) [2.5 mmol/l (96 mg/dl)] and British Hypertension Society (2004) [2.0 mmol/l (80 mg/dl)] guidelines (for details see Mikhailidis et al.[2]). Therefore, this patient needed cholesterol-lowering therapy. Given the previous reactions to statins, we started him on ezetimibe (10 mg/day), a selective inhibitor of intestinal cholesterol absorption.[2] Six weeks later the patient was tolerating ezetimibe very well. His CK, and renal and liver function remained normal. His LDL-cholesterol decreased from 4.2 to 3.1 mmol/l (162 to 120 mg/dl), representing a decrease of 26.2% (Table 1). However, we still had not achieved the LDL-cholesterol goals (see above). The options available were as follows:

(a) *Intensify therapeutic lifestyle changes (TLC)*. Weight loss, regular exercise, and diet could help achieve a small reduction in LDL-cholesterol levels. Furthermore, the addition of plant sterol/stanol supplements could further decrease the LDL-cholesterol concentration. To our knowledge, there are no studies assessing the combined effect of ezetimibe and plant sterols/stanols.
(b) *Add a fibrate*: this would further decrease triglycerides and increase HDL-cholesterol levels. However, only a 'small' reduction in LDL-cholesterol

176

levels would be anticipated. Moreover, the safety and efficacy of adding a fibrate to ezetimibe has not yet been established.[2]

(c) *Add nicotinic acid*: although nicotinic acid would further improve triglyceride and HDL-cholesterol levels, its effect on LDL-cholesterol levels is weaker than that of higher doses of statins. Furthermore, the safety and efficacy of adding nicotinic acid to ezetimibe has not been established.[2] Treatment with nicotinic acid could also adversely influence insulin sensitivity.

(d) *Increase the dose of OMACOR (concentrated omega-3 fish-oil esters)*: This could further reduce triglyceride levels but would not influence LDL-cholesterol or HDL-cholesterol concentrations.

(e) *Add a low-dose of a statin not previously tried by this patient*: Fluvastatin is associated with the smallest number of reported cases of statin-associated rhabdomyolysis and a frequency of CK elevation comparable with that seen with placebo, with no dose-related increases.[3] When several fluvastatin studies were evaluated, the incidence of CK elevation ($\geq 5\times$ the upper limit of the reference range) was 0.9%, 0.8%, 1.0%, and 0.3% for placebo and fluvastatin 20 mg, 40 mg, and extended-release (ER) 80 mg, respectively.[3] The incidence of a greater CK elevation ($\geq 10\times$ the upper limit of the reference range) was 0.2%, 0.2%, 0.3%, and 0% for placebo and fluvastatin 20 mg, 40 mg, and ER 80 mg, respectively. The rate (cases/10^6 prescriptions) of statin-related fatal rhabdomyolysis was reported as 0.04 for atorvastatin, 3.16 for cerivastatin (now withdrawn from the market), 0.00 for fluvastatin, 0.19 for lovastatin, 0.04 for pravastatin, and 0.12 for simvastatin.[3] Furthermore, fluvastatin has an evidence base. More specifically, the Lescol Intervention Prevention Study (LIPS) demonstrated that fluvastatin (80 mg/day) significantly reduced the risk of major adverse cardiac events (cardiac death, nonfatal MI, coronary artery bypass grafting or repeat PCI) by 22% as compared with placebo ($p=0.01$) in patients who underwent their first PCI.[3] This result was independent of baseline total cholesterol levels.

We decided to prescribe fluvastatin 20 mg/day together with TLC. Two months later the patient was doing well on fluvastatin (20 mg/day) plus ezetimibe (10 mg/day). His CK remained within the reference range and he was asymptomatic. The LDL-cholesterol dropped to 2.5 mmol/l (96 mg/dl) (Table 1), representing a 19.3% decrease from the previous value. The total decrease in LDL-cholesterol with the combined ezetimibe and low-dose fluvastatin treatment was 40.5%. As already stated, in view of the PCI and previous MI we should strive to lower his LDL-cholesterol to a value closer to 2.0 mmol/l (80 mg/dl). Therefore, we cautiously increased the dose of fluvastatin to 40 mg/day. Two months later the patient was still asymptomatic with a LDL-cholesterol of 2.3 mmol/l (89 mg/dl). This represents a further 7% reduction with doubling of the dose of the statin. In view of the previous statin-related muscle problems we felt that it was safer not to increase fluvastatin to 80 mg/day. The patient is currently doing well, with an acceptable LDL-cholesterol level of 2.1 mmol/l (81 mg/dl). We will consider increasing the dose of fluvastatin to 80 mg (ER formulation) per day if his LDL-cholesterol rises above the current value.

Comments

Although statins are safe drugs, some patients develop adverse effects (e.g. myopathy) that limit their use. This represents a major clinical problem when lipid-lowering therapy is mandatory. We now have alternative nonstatin hypolipidemic drugs in our armamentarium; ezetimibe is one of them. Ezetimibe can be used as monotherapy in patients who cannot tolerate statins or in combination therapy with a low dose of a statin, obviating the need for higher doses that may be associated with an increase in side effects.

All statins are not the same. Careful administration of a different statin may be undertaken in patients who are intolerant of other statins.

References

1. Grundy SM, Cleeman JI, Merz CNB et al. Implications of recent clinical trials for the national cholesterol education program adult treatment panel IIII guidelines. Circulation 2004; 110: 227–39.
2. Mikhailidis DP, Wierzbicki AS, Daskalopoulou SS et al. The use of ezetimibe in achieving low density lipoprotein lowering goals in clinical practice: position statement of a United Kingdom consensus panel. Curr Med Res Opin 2005; 21: 959–69.
3. Liberopoulos EN, Daskalopoulou SS, Mikhailidis DP, Wierzbicki AS, Elisaf MS. A review of the lipid-related effects of fluvastatin. Curr Med Res Opin 2005; 21: 231–43.

Case 35

STATIN INTOLERANCE IN A PATIENT FOLLOWING A KIDNEY TRANSPLANT

D John Betteridge

Case history

A 65-year-old man of Asian extraction was referred to the Lipid Clinic with a history of intolerance of statin therapy.

Originally from South Africa, he developed bilharzia due to *Schistosoma haematobium*; he attributed this to the necessity of swimming across rivers during his urgent escape from that country during less-enlightened times.

He developed chronic kidney failure and eventually required end-stage support. After 3 years of hemodialysis he received a successful kidney transplant at the age of 54 years.

At the age of 65 years he was admitted with acute coronary syndrome and underwent coronary angioplasty with stenting. He was discharged on simvastatin 40 mg/day for lipid lowering.

When seen for review he reported that he had stopped the drug because of marked generalized muscle pains and tenderness. The importance of statin therapy was re-emphasized to him as part of the secondary prevention of coronary disease and pravastatin 40 mg/day was prescribed.

After several weeks he developed similar symptoms and stopped the pravastatin. Five days later when he attended his primary care physician his creatine phosphokinase (CPK) was elevated at 856 IU/l.

He was referred to the Lipid Clinic for further advice because of his problems with statin therapy. On examination there was an arcus but no other signs of hyperlipidemia His BMI was 24.5, blood pressure was 127/83. He had no symptoms referable to the cardiovascular system.

Fasting lipid profile was as follows: total cholesterol 6.7 mmol/l, total triglyceride 2.7 mmol/l, HDL-cholesterol 0.9 mmol/l, LDL-cholesterol 4.6 mmol/l, apoprotein B 1.36 g/l, apoprotein A1 1.12 g/l, lipoprotein (a) 0.67 g/l. In addition, fasting glucose was 5.9 mmol/l, liver function tests were unremarkable, thyroid function was normal, and plasma creatinine was 160 μmol/l. Creatine phosphokinase was 190 IU/l.

179

Learning points

Kidney impairment, dyslipidemia, and increased cardiovascular disease (CVD) risk.
Dyslipidemia is common in chronic kidney disease and is characterized by
hypertriglyceridemia, low HDL-cholesterol, and increased concentrations of
lipoprotein (a). In addition there is also accumulation of atherogenic remnant
particles. The mechanisms are not fully understood. Hemodialysis can exacerbate
the hypertriglyceridemia through effects on lipoprotein lipase and its major co-
factor apoprotein CII. Lipoprotein (a) consists of an LDL particle to which is
attached a further apoprotein, apo a. This protein has close structural homology
with plasminogen and may influence fibrinolysis. It is a risk factor for CVD when
cholesterol levels are increased. It is likely that these lipid and lipoprotein
abnormalities contribute to the increased risk of CVD in chronic kidney disease.
In general the dyslipidemia improves following renal transplantation but in about a
quarter of patients it persists, possibly in relation to immunosuppressant therapy
(corticosteroids, cyclosporin), and weight gain among other factors.

Statin drug interactions. The clinical history was highly suggestive of myositis
associated with statin therapy. This conclusion was supported by the finding of an
elevated CPK taken a few days after stopping the statin.

This is a very rare but important complication of statin therapy and it
demonstrates an important practice point, which is to warn all patients to stop the
drug in the event of generalized, painful, tender muscles, often accompanied by
fatigue. This is important as rhabdomyolysis may develop if the drug is continued.

In this patient the concurrent long-term immunosuppressant therapy which
included cyclosporin had not been taken into account in the protocol-led
prescription of medicines following his emergency admission with coronary disease.

It is important to consider the possibility of drug interactions when prescribing
statins just as with any other drug class. With the exception of pravastatin all
statins are extensively metabolized by the cytochrome P450 (CYP) enzyme
system. Cyclosporin interferes with statin metabolism at CYP P450, increasing
plasma levels and consequently toxic potential. Cyclosporin is an inhibitor of
CYP3A4, which is important in the metabolism of simvastatin, lovastatin, and
atorvastatin. Other important drugs that can interact at CYP 3A4 are protease
inhibitors; erythromycin; the antifungal drugs ketoconazole, itraconazole, and
fluconazole; amiodarone, diltiazem, verapamil, and some antidepressants.

Fluvastatin (mainly metabolized through CYP2C9) and pravastatin (eliminated
by other metabolic routes) are unlikely to be affected by inhibition of CYP3A4.
However, another possible site of interaction between statins and cyclosporin has
been identified, namely P-glycoproteins, a newly recognized class of active drug
transporters. Atorvastatin, lovastatin, pravastatin, and simvastatin have been
identified as substrates and inhibitors of P-glycoprotein.

180

Although a small increase in the bioavailability of fluvastatin has been demonstrated with concomitant cyclosporin therapy, no episodes of increased CPK or muscle symptoms were reported in a large endpoint study in renal transplant patients. In this multicenter, double-blind, placebo-controlled trial 2102 renal transplant recipients with a total cholesterol of 4.0–9.0 mmol/l received fluvastatin (40 mg/day increased to 80 mg/day after 2 years), which reduced LDL-cholesterol by 32.5% at the end of the study (Holdass et al 2003).

Although the primary composite endpoint (including coronary interventions) was not significant there was a significant reduction in cardiac deaths and nonfatal MI. Importantly, rates of adverse events were similar in the fluvastatin and placebo groups. Greater than fivefold increases in CPK did not occur more commonly in the active treatment group and there were was no reported increase in myalgia.

There were two cases of rhabdomyolysis in the trial, one in each group, and both were related to severe trauma.

This clinical trial experience is encouraging and fluvastatin is the author's first choice statin in patients taking cyclosporin.

Summary

Chronic kidney disease is associated with dyslipidemia, which is likely to contribute significantly to the observed increase in CVD risk. Statins have an important role in reducing vascular risk in this population, as demonstrated from subgroup analyses of major statin trials. Post transplant patients are likely to be taking cyclosporin among other drugs and caution is necessary in the prescribing of statins that may be subject to important interactions at CYP450 3A4 or P-glycoprotein. Fluvastatin appears to be a safer alternative to consider in this situation.

Further reading

Baigent C, Burbury K, Wheeler D. Premature cardiovascular disease in chronic renal failure. Lancet 2000; 356: 147–52.

Ballantyne CM, Corsini A, Davidson MH et al. Risk for myopathy with statin therapy in high risk patients. Arch Intern Med 2003; 163: 553–64.

Bolego C, Baetta R, Bellosta S, Corsini A, Paoletti R. Safety considerations for statins. Curr Opin Lipidol 2002; 13: 637–44.

Holdaas H, Fellstrom B, Jardine AG et al. Effect of fluvastatin on cardiac outcomes in renal transplant recipients: a multicentre, randomised, placebo-controlled trial. Lancet 2003; 361: 2024–31.

Lindholm A, Albrechtsen D, Frodin L et al. Ischemic heart disease: a major cause of death and graft loss after renal transplantation in Scandinavia. Transplantation 1995; 60: 451–7.

Roodnat JI, Mulder PG, Zietse R et al. Cholesterol is an independent predictor of outcome after renal transplantation. Transplantation 2000; 69: 1704–10.

INDEX

N.B. Pages in italic denote material in tables of figures, but not in main text on that page.

A to Z trial 30–1
  design features/end-points *31*
abdominal pain 59–63
ACE inhibitors 76, 127
acipimox 51
acute coronary syndrome 29–33, 179
Adult Treatment Panel III (ATP-III)
  report 56
albuminuria 134–5, *136*
  as intervention target 136
alcohol abuse 125
alcohol consumption 123, 124–5
  and triglyceride levels 150
alcoholic fatty liver disease 124
amlodipine 15, 17, 26
angina 37
  exertional 7
  stable 51
  unstable 23
antilipotoxic drugs 101
apheresis *see* LDL apheresis
apolipoproteins *129*
  analysis 111
apolipoprotein B
  familial combined hyperlipidemia
    90, 110–11
  measurement 109–11
  as therapeutic target 32
  and thyroxine therapy 120
apolipoprotein B/apolipoprotein A1
  ratio 111
apolipoprotein B gene mutations
  35, 36, 39, 53
apolipoprotein E gene 65
apoprotein E 106

apoprotein E Leiden 107
Arterial Biology for Investigation
    of Treatment Effects of Reducing
    Cholesterol (ARBITER)-2
  study 168
aspirin 7
  CHD 16, 24
  dyslipidemia 175
  familial hypercholesterolemia
    37, 166
  triglyceridemia 57
atenolol 7, 15, 16, 131, 132, 175
atherogenic dyslipidemia 20
atherosclerosis
  dyslipidemias 159
  familial combined
    hyperlipidemia 111
  familial hypercholesterolemia
    35, 42
  family history of 86
  hypercholesterolemic patients'
    offspring 45
  hyperlipoproteinemia type III 107
  hypothyroidism 115
atorvastatin 9, 11, 12, 16
  acute coronary syndrome 30, 32
  diabetes 138
  dominant hypercholesterolemia *52*
  familial combined
    hyperlipidemia 95
  familial hypercholesterolemia 35,
    37, 39, *40*, 166, *167*, 168
  and glomerular filtration rate 135
  intolerance to 175
  lipemia 105

metabolic syndrome 145, 172
metabolism 180
Atorvastatin-Simvastatin
	Atherosclerosis Prevention
	(ASAP) 168
Atromid (clofibrate) *see* clofibrate
	(Atromid)

beta-blockers 24, 37
bezafibrate 51, *52*, 105
bile acid sequestrants 21, 51, 54, 56
bilharzia 179
biliary obstruction 47, 49
bisoprolol 24, 26
'bright liver' 99
British Hypertension Society
	guidelines 15
broad beta disease 106

Camelot trial 17
cardiovascular risk
	apolipoproteins 112
	assessment of individual 17
	hepatic lipase/LDL-cholesterol 20
	and insulin resistance 80, *82*
	and metabolic syndrome 80
	reduced with statins 8
	scoring systems 56
	and subclinical hypothyroidism 119
	in triglyceridemia 56
'cardiovascular time bomb' 100
CARDS 30, 129, 138
CARE trial 30
cerivastatin 33
CHAMP study 30
CHD *see* coronary heart disease
	(CHD)
children
	familial hypercholesterolemia 38
	hypercholesterolemia 51
	hypertriglyceridemia, severe 65

cholesterol absorption inhibitors
	41–2
	site of action 41
	with statins 41
Cholesterol and Recurrent Events
	(CARE) trial 138
cholesterol levels
	increasing during pregnancy 44
	during LDL apheresis 44
	see also HDL-cholesterol levels;
		LDL-cholesterol levels;
		serum cholesterol levels
cholesterol synthesis/absorption 41–2
cholestyramine 35
	dominant hypercholesterolemia *52*
	familial combined
		hyperlipidemia 95
	familial hypercholesterolemia
		39, *40*
	xanthomatous neuropathy 47, 48
chylomicrons 60, 61
	clearance 88, *89*
	familial LPL deficiency 67
chylomicron particles 148
chylomicronemia 65, 148
chylomicronemia syndrome 148
clofibrate (Atromid) 105, 107
	side effects 107
clopidogrel 24, 37, 175
colestipol 43, 51, *52*
Collaborative Atorvastatin
	Diabetes Study (CARDS)
	30, 129, 138
combination therapy 95
	complex dyslipidemia 159–63
	familial hypercholesterolemia 37,
		38, 39, 96–8
	in two brothers *167*
	hyperlipidemia 153–7, 165–9
	hypertriglyceridemia 151
	lipid-lowering 7–10

metabolic syndrome 145, 156
side effects 156
combined hyperlipidemia
72–112
ethanol-induced 123–6
treatments available 153
see also familial combined
hyperlipidemia
corneal arcus 35, 36, 39, 51,
166, 171
coronary artery bypass graft
(CABG) 7, 11, 16, 51, *52*
coronary artery disease 7
reducing risk 8
coronary heart disease (CHD)
diabetes 23–7
mortality rates 24
dyslipidemia 175–8
patients 15–33
high-risk 1–5, 74
moderate-risk 1–5
multiple risk factor 11–13
younger females 15, 16–17
reducing risk 1–5
risk factors 1, 5, 12
intensive management 27
multiple 1–13
screening of family members 100
coronary risk prediction by
JBS 1, 2–3
cyclosporin 95
drug interactions 180, 181

Diabetes Atherosclerosis Intervention
Study (DAIS) 137
diabetes mellitus, type II 80, 127–30,
131–42
and acute coronary
syndrome 29–33
cholesterol increase in 127
combination therapy for 153

complicating
hypercholesterolemia 12
and coronary heart disease 23–7
mortality rates 24
early intervention 138–9
with fatty liver disease 99–103
and hypertension 131, 132
lipid-lowering therapy 129
menopausal woman 153–4
renoprotective interventions 136
risk factors/adverse effects 136
testing for 133
triglyceridemia 62
younger patients 129
diabetic dyslipidemia 128, 132–4
management 128–30
diabetic ketoacidosis 59, 60
diabetic kidney disease
(nephropathy) 133–7
assessment of severity 134
and metformin 137
testing for 134
urinary tract infection
confounding diagnosis 134
diet
complex dyslipidemia 161
diabetes 24, 127, 130
familial combined hyperlipidemia
90
familial LPL deficiency 69–70
high LDL-cholesterol 2, 5
hyperlipidemia 62
metabolic syndrome
74, 156, 172
dry skin 117–21
dysbetalipoproteinemia 106
see also familial
dysbetalipoproteinemia
dyslipidemias
combined, management of 76
complex 159–63, 175–8

diabetic 128, 132–4
  management 128–30
  with fatty liver disease 99–103
  with metabolic syndrome 73,
    79–83
    management steps 76
    therapy 80–2
  and polycystic ovary syndrome 21
  as risk factor for diabetic
    nephropathy 135
  secondary 113–51
  severe 35–72
  and statin intolerance 180

ectopic lipid accumulation
  insulin resistance 100–1
  insulin sensitivity 101
endocannabinoid receptor blockers 24
erythromycin with statins 95
estrogen
  in hypertriglyceridemia 150
  masking lipid disorders 19, 20
  see also hormone replacement
    therapy
ethanol consumption 123, 124–5
  see also alcohol abuse; ethanol
    consumption
ethnicity
  and CHD 16
  and hypertension 15
EUROASPIRE 2 27
exercise
  diabetes 24, 99, 130
  familial combined
    hyperlipidemia 90
  high LDL-cholesterol 2, 5
  metabolic syndrome 172
  triglyceridemia 57, 58
exercise stress tests 16, 23
ezetimibe 12, 39, 40, 42
  dominant hypercholesterolemia
    51, 52, 54

dyslipidemia 176
  familial combined
    hyperlipidemia 96
  familial hypercholesterolemia
    166, 167
  metabolic syndrome 76
  with statins 97, 98, 168, 177
  thyroiditis 118

familial atherosclerosis
    treatment study (FATS)
    168–9
familial combined hyperlipidemia
    12, 85–91, 110–11
  clinical features 89
  diagnosis 86, 88
  differential diagnosis 86, 87
  features 110
  genetics 86
  and insulin resistance 90
  management 95–8
  metabolic features 88, 89
  metabolic syndrome,
    similarity to 89
  prevalence 110
  therapy 89
  treatment 90–1
familial dysbetalipoproteinemia 86
  autosomal dominant 87
  differential diagnosis 87
familial hypercholesterolemia
    (FH) 35, 39–42, 110
  clinical phenotype, patient
    with 35–8
  combination therapy 165
  family screening 169
  hypothyroidism 113–16
    autoimmune 115
    family tree 114
  laboratory investigations 157
  timing of treatment 38
  treatment 157

familial hypertriglyceridemia 86
  differential diagnosis 87
familial LPL deficiency
  breastfeeding in 70
  pedigree chart 67
  in pregnancy 65–72
fatty liver disease *see* alcoholic
    fatty liver disease;
    non-alcoholic fatty liver
    disease
fenofibrate 33, 59, 145
  complex dyslipidemia 161
  diabetes 137
  hypertriglyceridemia 150
  pancreatitis 60
  statins 32, 75, 98
  triglyceridemia 57
Fenofibrate Intervention and
    Event Lowering in
    Diabetes Study 129
fetal status
  HELP therapy 43
  hypercholesterolemia 44–5
FH *see* familial hypercholesterolemia
fibrates 13, 56, 58
  adverse effects 137, 153
  diabetes 129, 137
  dyslipidemia 176–7
  hypertriglyceridemia 150
  metabolic syndrome 76, 81,
    82, 144
  with statins 97, *145*, 156
  triglyceridemia 62
fish oil 8, 13, 56
  dyslipidemia 175, 177
  problems with 162–3
  triglyceridemia 62
floating beta disease 106
fluvastatin 177–8, 180, 181
  bioavailability 181
4S trial 30, 75, 138, 168
Framingham risk score 56

gemfibrozil 11, 13, 32, 33
  adverse effects 58
  diabetes 137
  familial combined
    hyperlipidemia 95
  hyperlipoproteinemia
    type III 107
  hypertriglyceridemia 150
  and insulin resistance 81, *82*
genetics
  autosomal dominant
    hypercholesterolemia 53–4
  chylomicronemia 148
  familial combined
    hyperlipidemia 86
  familial hypercholesterolemia
    35, 36, 38
  familial LPL deficiency 69
  hepatic lipase 20
  hyperchylomicronemia 61, 66
  hyperlipoproteinemia type III 107
glipizide 160
glitazones 91
glycemic control 130
  hypertriglyceridemia 133, 137
glyceryl trinitrate 15
gout 73, 75, 77
GREek Atorvastatin/Coronary heart
    disease Evaluation (GREACE)
    study 135

HDL-cholesterol levels
  and alcohol consumption 125
  coronary heart disease 1
  increasing 5, 8, 9, 160
  metabolic syndrome 75, 144
  and statins 33
heart healthy diet 5
Heart Outcomes Prevention
    Evaluation (HOPE) trial 26
Heart Protection Study (HPS)
    26, 30, 75, 129, 135

187

Helsinki Heart Study 129, 137
hemodialysis 180
heparin-induced extracorporeal LDL
        precipitation (HELP) therapy
    post-delivery 44
    during pregnancy 43
hepatic lipase 19, 20, 21, *162*
    genetic polymorphisms 20
hepatic steatosis 73
high-density lipoprotein-cholesterol
        levels *see* HDL-cholesterol levels
HMG-CoA reductases *see* statins
hormone replacement therapy
        150, 156–7
hydrochlorothiazide 160
hypercholesterolemia 1–5, 11–13
    autosomal dominant 51–4
        family tree *52*
        features 53
        response to therapy *52*
    in child 51
    with hypothyroidism 115
    polygenic 113
    severe 154
    see also familial
            hypercholesterolemia
hyperchylomicronemia 61
    genetics 66
    pedigree chart 67
    serum sample 67
hyperlipidemia
    combination therapy 153–7
        triple therapy 165–9
    treatments available 153
    see also combined hyperlipidemia;
            familial combined
            hyperlipidemia
hyperlipoproteinemia 60
    classification 60–1
    with metabolic syndrome 73–7
    type I 60, 66

type III 60, 106
    biochemistry/pathogenesis
        106–7
    features 107
    genetics 107
    treatment 107–8
type IV 60
type V 60–1
hypertension 15, 73
    lipid-neutral agents 150
    management 76
    and subclinical hypothyroidism
        118–19
hypertriglyceridemia
        12, 55–8, 62
    with acute pancreatitis
        60, 62, 70
        mortality/morbidity 68
    acute pancreatitis, avoidance of 150
    clinical features 148, 149–50
    diabetes 128
    ethanol-induced 123
    and ischemic heart disease 62
    management 150–1
    maternal 65, 70
        management 69
    postmenopausal woman 147–51
    secondary causes *149*
        treatment for 150–1
    severe 13
hyperuricemia 73, 74
hypoalphalipoproteinemia 165
hypothyroidism
    autoimmune 115
    diabetes 128
    with hypercholesterolemia 114–15
    increasing statin side-effects 175
    see also subclinical hypothyroidism

indapamide 16
insulin 59, 60

insulin resistance 73, 80, 155
    combination therapy for 153
    with dyslipidemia 161
        therapy 80–2
    and 'ectopic' lipid 100–1
    with fatty liver disease 99–103
    and liposuction 101
    management 76
insulin sensitizing therapy 82, 91, 161
INTERHEART 111
intrahepatic lipid content 100

Joint British Societies (JBS) coronary
    risk prediction 1, 2–3

ketoacidosis 59, 60
kidney transplant, statin intolerance
    after 179–82

lansoprazole 175
LDL apheresis 36, 38, 39, 40, 45
    for dominant
        hypercholesterolemia 54
    during pregnancy 43–6
        results 44
    see also heparin-induced
        extracorporeal LDL
        precipitation (HELP) therapy
LDL-cholesterol levels
    as CHD risk 1–2
    in diabetes 133
    familial hypercholesterolemia 35
    in familial hypercholesterolemia 37
    and fish oil 13
    goals in dyslipidemia 176
    guidelines in CHD patients 8
    in hypercholesterolemia with
        hypothyroidism 115
    lowering 8–9
    targets 32
    therapy for high levels 2, 3, 5

LDL metabolism in diabetes 133
LDL particles 12, 19, 20
    clearance, reduced 110–11, 119
    in diabetes 133
    in familial combined hyperlipidemia
        110–11
    lowering numbers 21
    as therapeutic target 32
left anterior descending artery
    stenosis 24
Lescol Intervention Prevention Study
    (LIPS) 177
lifestyle modification 8, 24
    in dyslipidemia 176
    in familial combined
        hyperlipidemia 90
    in hyperlipidemia 62
    in metabolic syndrome 74, 75,
        77, 144, 145, 156, 171–3
    in pancreatitis 60
lipemia 172
    postprandial 132
    see also mixed lipemia
lipemia retinalis 59, 60, 66, 149
lipid-lowering therapy
    and cardiovascular events 30
    combination 7–10, 37,
        38, 39, 96–8
    and diabetic nephropathy 135
    evidence of success 30
    familial combined
        hyperlipidemia 90
    high LDL-cholesterol 2, 3, 5, 30
    metabolic syndrome 156
    peripheral arterial disease 144
    reducing diabetes risk 136
lipid profiles
    acute coronary syndrome 179
    with atorvastatin 12
    before/after alcohol
        withdrawal 124

before/after thyroxine therapy *118*
with combined therapy 39, *40*
complex dyslipidemia 160
diabetes *129*
   after treatment 26
   uncontrolled 24
dyslipidemias before/after
    therapy *176*
effects of combination therapy *145*
familial hypercholesterolemia 166
   two brothers *167*
after fibrate therapy 151
hyperlipoproteinemia type III 106
inter-individual variations *88*
and nicotinic acid 11
with simvastatin +/- niacin 8
timing of measurement 30
xanthomatous neuropathy 48
LIPID trial 30
lipoprotein (a), therapy for 168, 169
lipoprotein catabolism *162*
lipoprotein lipase (LPL) 69
   activation 161
   and alcohol consumption 125
   deficiency 69
    genetics 69
    pedigree chart *67*
    during pregnancy 65–72
   triglycerides, effect on *162*
lipoprotein metabolism in
   diabetes 128
lipoprotein particles 110–11
   see also LDL particles
liporegulation 101
liposuction and insulin resistance 101
lisinopril 15
liver disease *see* non-alcoholic fatty
   liver disease
liver function
   before/after alcohol
    withdrawal *124*

and combined therapy 77
metabolic syndrome 101
and statins 9, 10, 50
lovastatin (mevinolin) 11
metabolism 180
triglyceridemia 58
xanthomatous neuropathy 47, 48
low-density lipoprotein-cholesterol
   levels *see* LDL-cholesterol levels
Lp-X 48, 49
LPL *see* lipoprotein lipase (LPL)
LT4 therapy *see* thyroxine (LT4)
   therapy
luminal irregularities, arterial
   24, *25*

macrolides with statins 96
metabolic syndrome (syndrome X)
   12, 19, 80, 155
   as CHD marker 100
   and diabetes 74
   with dyslipidemia 73, 79–83
    management steps 76
    therapy 80–2
   with hyperlipoproteinemia 73–7
   lifestyle modification, impact
    of 171–3
   and peripheral arterial disease
    143–6
    management 144
    treatment options 144–5
   therapy 13
metformin 26, 76, 127, 137, 160,
   172
metoprolol 160
milky serum 55, 59, *60*
mixed lipemia 105–8
myositis
   in combination therapy
    153, 156
   statin-induced 96, 108

National Cholesterol Education
Program (NCEP) Adult
Treatment Panel III (ATP-III)
report 56, 80, 129, 144,
176
nephropathy, diabetic *see* diabetic
kidney disease (nephropathy)
NHANES III study 116, 134
niacin 9
  combined with statins 9–10
  complex dyslipidemia 160
  and diabetes control 13
  extended-release 9
  familial combined
      hyperlipidemia 95
  familial hypercholesterolemia
      166, *167*, 168
  hypertriglyceridemia 150
  and insulin resistance 137–8
  for lowering triglycerides 56, 57
  in metabolic syndrome 81
  side effects 9, 57, 153
  with statins 97, 156
  in triglyceridemia 58
Niaspan 160, 166
  with statins 98
nicotinic acid 11, 13, 166
  dominant hypercholesterolemia 51
  dyslipidemia 177
  familial hypercholesterolemia
      37, 39, *40*
  triglyceridemia 62
nitroglycerin 29
non-alcoholic fatty liver
      disease (NAFLD)
      99–103, 150
  features *101*
  hepatic fat, origins of 101
  prevalence *101*
  reversal by weight loss 100
nutritional control *see* diet

obesity
  and insulin resistance 80
  with metabolic syndrome 76
OMACOR 175, 177
oral contraceptives 21
  for familial hypercholesterolemia 37
  masking lipid disorders 19
orlistat 163
osteoarthropathy 47
oxazepam 23

P-glycoproteins 180
'P' program 2
  statins 2, 3, 4–5
pancreatitis 56
  acute 59–63, 65
      and alcohol consumption 125
      avoidance 150
      with hypertriglyceridemia
          60, 68
      mortality/morbidity 68
  chylomicronemia-associated
      149, 150
  in combined hyperlipidemias *87*
  and hormone replacement
      therapy 157
PCSK9 gene mutations 53–4
D-penicillinamine 47
percutaneous transluminal
      interventions 37
perindopril 16, 77
peripheral arterial
      disease (PAD)
  aggressive risk factor
      modification 145
  and metabolic syndrome
      143–6
  management 144
  treatment options 144–5
physical activity *see* exercise
pioglitazone 161

plasma exchange 45
    combined with statins 48
    familial hypercholesterolemia 39
    serum cholesterol rebound
        48, *49*
    xanthomatous neuropathy
        47, 48
polycystic ovary syndrome
    (PCOS) 19, 21
pravastatin 21, 30
    intolerance to 175, 179
    metabolism 180
Pravastatin or Atorvastatin Evaluation
    and Infection Trial (PROVE-IT)
    see PROVE-IT
pre-conception counseling 69
PREVENT study 168
propranolol 23
PROVE-IT 26, 168
    TIMI 22 30, 31
        design features/end-points *31*
        LDL-cholesterol target levels 32
pseudohyponatremia 61–2

ramipril 26, 160, 175
remnant particle disease 106
renal function, impaired
    diabetic nephropathy 133–7
    increasing statin side-effects 175
renal transplant, statin intolerance
    after 179–82
renin–angiotensin system 136
reverse cholesterol transport
    (RCT) 20
rosuvastatin 21
    dominant hypercholesterolemia 51
    familial hypercholesterolemia
        37, 39, *40*

Scandinavian Simvastatin Survival
    Study (4S) 30, 75, 138, 168

serum cholesterol levels
    familial hypercholesterolemia 35
    post plasma exchange rebound
        48, *49*
simvastatin 3, 5, 7, 11
    acute coronary syndrome 30
    combination therapy
        with ezetimibe 12, 76
        with fenofibrate 75
    diabetes plus CHD 24, 27
    dyslipidemia, complex 160
    effect on lipid profile 8
    and glomerular filtration rate 135
    hypercholesterolemia 113–14
        dominant 51
        familial 39, *40*, 50, *167*, 168
    intolerance to 175, 179
    metabolism 180
    side effects 117
    triglyceridemia, extreme 55
spironolactone 47
statins (HMG-CoA reductases)
    acute coronary syndrome 30
    combination therapy 96–8, 145
        with cholesterol absorption
            inhibitors 41
        with cholestyramine 168
        with ezetimibe 97, 98, 168, 177
        with fenofibrate 32, 98
        with fibrates 97, *145*, 156
        with niacin 97, 156, 168
        with/without niacin 9–10
        with Niaspan 98
    diabetes 30, 128–9, 138
        with CHD 29
        with dyslipidemia 137
    drug interactions 180
    dyslipidemia 177
    first use in UK 50
    high cholesterol levels 79
    high LDL-cholesterol 2

hypercholesterolemia, dominant
51, 54
hyperlipoproteinemia
type III 107
hypertriglyceridemia 13, 151
hypothyroidism 116
intolerance to 175–8
after kidney transplant 179–82
and Lp-X levels 49
metabolic syndrome 76, 81,
82, 144–5
'pleiotropic effects' 138
side effects 5, 33, 97, 98,
116, 117
increased 175
limiting use 178
site of action 41
stopped in breastfeeding 44
stopped in pregnancy 43, 44
triglyceridemia 58
xanthomatous neuropathy 47
Steno-2 trial 27
stenosis
of coronary arteries 24, 25, 29
severe 16
stenting/stents 24, 25
drug-eluting 29, 32
subclinical hypothyroidism
117, 118
cardiovascular risk 119
and hypertension 118–19
patient selection 120
sulfonylureas 137
syndrome X see metabolic syndrome
(syndrome X)

tendon xanthomata 35, 39, 51,
154, 166
therapeutic issues 151–82
therapeutic lifestyle changes (TLC)
see lifestyle modification

thiazide 26, 150
thiazolidinedione (TZD) 82,
137, 161
thyroiditis, autoimmune 117
thyrotoxicosis 47
thyroxine (LT4) therapy 47,
115, 118
adverse effects 120
lipid effects 119–20
response to treatment 115
Treat to New Targets (TNT) study
9, 26, 32
triglyceride levels
and alcohol consumption 125
diabetes 133
management 137
and estrogen 19
familial combined
hyperlipidemia 86
familial LPL deficiency 68
and fish oil 13
lowering 8, 9, 81
metabolic syndrome 144
in pregnancy 68
triglyceridemia, extreme 55–8
triple therapy for hyperlipidemia
165–9
in two brothers 167

UK Prospective Diabetes Study
(UKPDS) 26
umbilical artery blood flow in
hypercholesterolemia 44–5
urate levels 73, 75, 77

very low-density lipoproteins
see VLDLs
Veterans Administration HDL
Intervention Trial (VA HIT)
32–3, 75, 129
on fibrates 81, 82, 137

vitamin supplementation 47
VLDLs 60
  and alcohol consumption 125
  diabetes 133
  familial LPL deficiency 67

weight control/loss 8, 26
  diabetes 24, 99, 130
  fatty liver disease reversal 100
  hyperlipidemia 62
  metabolic syndrome 74, 76, 172
    variability of effect 75
  polycystic ovary syndrome 21
West of Scotland Coronary Prevention
  Study (WOSCOPS) 74, 136

women
  and cardiovascular risk 19–22
  and CHD 15, 16–17
    multiple risk factors 11–13

xanthomata 39, 51, 106,
  154, 166
  eruptive 59–63, *60*, *108*, 149
    regression 151
  hyperlipoproteinemia type III 107
  palmar *108*
xanthomatous neuropathy 47–50
  investigations 48
  physical signs 47
  xanthomata in 48